UNBLOCK
YOUR BODY

How Decompressing Your Fascia Is the Missing Link
in Healing Edited by Shauna Hardy

DEANNA HANSEN
Certified Athletic Therapist, Founder of
Fluid Isometrics and Block Therapy

Foreword by Dr. John Daugherty

UNBLOCK YOUR BODY
Copyright © 2020 by Deanna Hansen

How Decompressing Your Fascia Is the Missing Link in Healing Edited by Shauna Hardy

For permissions contact:

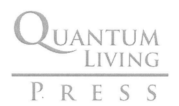

An Imprint for GracePoint Publishing (www.GracePointPublishing.com)
GracePoint Matrix, LLC 322 N Tejon St. #207 Colorado
Springs CO 80903 www.GracePointMatrix.com
Email: Admin@GracePointMatrix.com SAN # 991-6032

Library of Congress Control Number: *2020913520*
ISBN-13: (Paperback) #*978-1-951694-10-4*
eISBN: (eBook) # *978-1-951694-19-7*

Books may be purchased for educational, business, or sales promotional use.
For bulk order requests and price schedule contact: Orders@GracePointPublishing.com

Printed in the United States of America

Disclaimer

This books intended purpose is not to substitute the medical advice of a physician or qualified therapist. The reader should regularly consult a physician in matters relating to his/her health and particularly with respect to any symptoms that may require diagnosis or medical attention.

CONTENTS

FOREWORD

I have to admit that I am a bit of a fascia freak, so this book spoke to me. I was honored to write this foreword. I have been a longtime student and practitioner of research, methods and active practice working with the fascia system. I have always believed that healing is dependent on the confluence of the brain and nervous system, the many energy systems of the body and the ability to adapt and respond to our environment. I have worked with posture correction and postural balance, the treatment of athletic injuries and physical and emotional trauma in my everyday practice using the fascia system as my main focus of therapy. I firmly believe that the fascia system is one of the most essential communication systems for the Body-Mind.

I know from 35 plus years of clinical experience that emotions, pain, and trauma are stored in the fascia. When the right bodywork and specific intentional release methods are applied to the body, we can create enough space to restore the body's natural flow. It is then that the emotions, pain and trauma can be released from the body. When this occurs, as practitioners, we get the unique opportunity to see the body heal. We get to see the body right itself. Many times, that is experienced as the release of pain - chronic or acute. Many times, it is improved with more fluid posture and movement. Often, it is experienced as decreased muscle and overall body tension, a feeling of being at ease or an increase in a sense of wellbeing. Any author willing to write about how they have taken on healing the body through the fascia system not only needs to be heard, but should be honored and respected for their research, perseverance, and commitment. It has taken pioneers in the field like Ida Rolf, Thomas Meyers, Daniel Keown, John Barnes, and John Upledger, just to name a few, to transform the way we think about the body.

This book is a very exciting, entertaining, and compassionate account of the life work of a brilliant and talented woman on a mission. Deanna Hansen has taken the complex science concepts of the fascia system and her decades of hands on bodywork, posture correction and breathwork and created this book that guides us through self-help and self-care measures that we can practice for a lifetime.

In this stressful and competitive modern society, we have fostered body tension, pain, feelings of unworthiness, self-judgment, and loss of the sacred. The principles of Fluid Isometrics and Block Therapy articulated in Unblock Your Body is essential for reclaiming our wellness, a renewed relationship with your body, and living a joyful and liberated life.

In the process of evolving this work, Deanna has brought relief to countless clients who could not get help with their chronic pain, severe scoliosis, loss of function from injury, and recovery from surgery. She has helped countless clients improve their athletic performance and helped them love and appreciate their bodies into looking better and feeling better. In short, she has transformed their lives.

As you read this book, we will all be inspired by Deanna's touching stories of what appear to be "miraculous" healings; yet what Deanna shows us in this book is that we are all capable of experiencing such healing miracles. Renewal is built into the very fabric of our bodies. In truth, degeneration and disease are the exception, not the norm. Even though most of us have just accepted that aging, degeneration and disease are just the way it goes, once we understand how our bodies renew themselves, by creating space, inflating space and maintaining space in our fascia, we can harness these physiological processes intentionally.

With the use of Fluid Isometrics/Block Therapy, the fascia begins to change, the collagen and proteins begin to regenerate, and our cells get the oxygen, nutrients, blood flow, and waste removal essential to our wellness. Deanna teaches us that we can steer this process with intention, breath, and the Block. This allows us to put ourselves and our bodies back in the powerful position of driver in our transformation, rather than the passive role of passenger in our health and wellness.

A new generation of researchers coined a term for the renewal I have found in my own practice and that Deanna creates through Block Therapy called self-directed neuroplasticity or (SDN). The idea behind the term is that we direct the formation of new neural pathways and fascial fluidity. We also breakdown the old neuropathways and fascia constrictions through the quality of the experiences we cultivate. I am in total alignment that SDN will become one of the most potent and important concepts in personal transformation for the coming generation. I feel that this book will be at the forefront of that movement. Unblock your fascia, redirect neuroplasticity, change physiology, and change your life.

This valuable and easy to assimilate book will extend the reach of Deanna Hansen's remarkable contribution to bodywork and healing far and wide. I applaud her for taking the time from her already busy schedule of workshops, classes, courses, and active practice to write it all down for us. I hope you find Deanna's book, workshops, guidance, and instruction as enticing and exciting as I have.

Most importantly, Unblock Your Body reawakens us to the deepest aspects of our body - the fundamental balance, openness and essence of who we are. It returns us to the happiness and freedom that are the birthright of every human being. Read these pages slowly. Take their words and practices to heart. Let them guide you and create space for the expression of the best version of yourself in the world. Believe in your ability to realize your highest potential and take inspired action. Then you will become the unblocked true expression in the world that creates a happy and healthy future for yourself and for our planet.

Dr. John Daugherty, DC Author of *The Health Code*

THE STATE OF THE WORLD

We are living in interesting times. With the internet, there is exponential growth and creation, but also a greater awareness of the crises in life. As with everything, it is a double-edged sword. Negative information is the predominant theme of many messages shared with the masses and greed is their driver; we are all seemingly competing for something. This energy is causing many people to make choices from a place of fear rather than wisdom, and it is affecting the state of the world.

Who would have thought that a moment of intense fear would give birth to a system that would help many? But it has; the excitement is spreading about both Fluid Isometrics (the name of the therapeutic practice) and Block Therapy (the self-care form). For the past two decades, I have had the pleasure of working with tens of thousands of patients, either hands-on or through teaching new practitioners. It has been quite a ride and it feels like it's just beginning. As I write this, there are over 155 teachers throughout the world, either actively serving their community or in the process of learning these healing mechanisms.

For optimal health, the body needs balance and symmetry. A healthy body can withstand life's stresses as it has the ability to feed and clean itself properly.

Unfortunately, the collapsed posture — a physical manifestation of imbalance — is impairing this process and the detrimental results can be seen around the world. It is especially disturbingly evident in the young.

Anxiety and depression are also rampant among youth. This is creating a dynamic that we, as a collective, need to recognize. Our children are our future; yet, for the first time in human history, they will likely not survive their elders . . . unless something changes.

The key lies in the fascia system. This connective tissue literally encases every single cell in the body. It is ingenious in its design and exists to support as well as protect us, but it needs care and attention to function effectively.

Fortunately, there is a growing awareness in the scientific community of the importance of the fascia. In 2007, the world's first Fascia Conference was held in Boston, at Harvard University. In the advertisements, it stated that only about four percent of the tissue called fascia was understood. I was eager to attend and grateful for the experience; I realized I had a unique understanding of this tissue through my work and research.

Fluid Isometrics uses a practitioner's hands and other body parts (feet, knees, forearms, etc) to provide pressure that enables release of unnatural connective adhesions between cells and tissue or bone. Block Therapy enables you to achieve the same results on your own with a hand-finished cedar wooden block specifically designed to melt through layers of adhesion and scar tissue.

When it comes to fascia, our challenge is that it grips and seals to bone with tremendous magnetic force in order to counter the constant drag of gravity as well as maintain balance along with stability. The fascia follows a spiral pattern as this is how energy travels - in waves and spirals.

Fluid Isometrics and Block Therapy move into the spirals to release adhesions; this awakens cells previously blocked from flow and changes every aspect of your being. When you learn how to support your fascia, your body becomes more than just a physical container for survival. It becomes your means to thrive.

This applies to everyone. Anxiety, sleep issues, depression, chronic pain, mental suffering, scoliosis, toxic bodies . . . everything that is wrong with our health ties back to the fascia. Since that first conference in 2007, there has been mounting evidence to support this concept. I am pleased to be able to share my work and see it grow and evolve.

It seems that almost nothing in mainstream culture comes from a place of peace. Movies are full of violence and high-speed imagery; advertisers use fear to encourage us to buy their products; our technology bombards us with messages and information that we feel driven to stay on top of. The state of most things is chaotic and bullying is the tactic of those seemingly in charge. If you are paying attention to the media, you recognize that peace is not the message.

When you are afraid, your first reaction is to hold your breath; it is the natural response to pain, fear, and stress. In a situation of genuine threat, this would trigger the adrenal glands to send out hormones for the fight-or-flight response that provides an extra boost of energy — a necessary advantage in the face of danger.

However, in a world where it feels like danger is always lurking, breath is chronically restricted and the adrenal glands become exhausted.

Compensatory breathing muscles kick in for survival. Necessary oxygen gets inhaled, but it is hardly sufficient. This has fundamentally altered our physiology. Our fascia in particular has become frozen, dry, compressed, and toxic. We have become dense and dirty. Our movements are labored and lumbering, not flowing with grace and ease.

A healthy cell requires space both around and inside it. Restriction impairs function. Think of how you feel in a crammed elevator. Someone's cologne is oppressive, somebody else is talking too loud, you are getting squished into a corner — all in all, you feel miserable. As soon as the doors open and you are able to escape, you take a deep breath and luxuriate in the space around you. Your well-being is restored.

Your body is composed of trillions of cells, each with a specific function. Every cell is a universe in and of itself. The beauty, synchronicity, and mystery of cellular intelligence is mind blowing, but it all relies on space.

If something goes wrong with the cells, western-style medical practitioners will run tests to see if anything is lacking or depleted; then they will put into the body whatever is missing in the form of prescription medication. Unfortunately, this doesn't give the cells what they actually need: room to breathe. The body knows what it requires to heal from stress or trauma; our responsibility is to ensure that our cells have sufficient space to provide smooth passage for blood, oxygen, and nutrients as well as waste removal.

We can enhance these cellular missions with proper posture and breathing. If postural support is weak, the overall structure suffers. If the breath is weak, the cells deflate like a balloon losing air. Properly aligned and oxygenated cells are magnetized and energized. With this, cellular communication flows easily, and the body is able to respond appropriately where protection and support are most needed.

Today, most people have weak foundations and poor breathing habits. The fascia responds by degenerating from a natural resting place to getting sucked into collapsing structures and building dense floors and walls. Chronic compression of space reduces blood flow — everything gets colder, dirtier, and stickier.

It's a vicious cycle.

No wonder we are anxious.

Though the overall picture seems dark, there is hope. The relentless bleakness that the media disseminate is not the whole story.

For one thing, our fascia can change for the better. We are not confined to our current state of physical and psychological being. We have the power to unlock our dense bodies and breathe life into them. What we have been told about the inevitability of aging is also only a fraction of the story.

There is hope for adults and young persons alike. Today's youth are engaged in a life and death struggle. Computer postural syndrome is causing an accelerating collapse in their bodies. It doesn't help that from the start they are breathing from the wrong place.

People of my generation began life breathing from the belly. You could see this in healthy babies - the belly would rise and fall with breathing. Over time, pain, fear, and stress led to reactive breath holding and the compensatory muscles of the upper chest took over. In essence, we started life as effective breathers, but that changed.

Today, the newborn starts with a collapsed posture. Children are already breathing with the upper chest in their developmental years. Their physiology is already compromised as the most important nutrient — oxygen — is simply not as available to the cells as it should be. Like being in the crammed elevator, the cells are under stress. The body adapts, but there is only energy to survive, not to thrive.

By recognizing these essential needs for space and structure, we can embark on restoring health to our lives. The fascia can change. This remarkable tissue that connects and embraces every cell in the body wants to thrive; it wants to be open and spacious and free to function. When cells have room to be properly fed and cleaned, there is no anxiety. Once your cells are relaxed, you can actually live.

So you can see there is a connection between physical space and our mental place. This is a fundamental inspiration behind all of my work. That revelation was my discovery of the vital significance of the fascia in all matters of physical and psychological health.

Pain is a necessary part of our growth, but suffering is not. When you take your fascia health into your own hands and become your own health-care practitioner, you begin to shape your future as opposed to letting gravity take you down, slowly, steadily, day by day. Join me now as we look more deeply into how you can do this, and the repercussions of taking these healing steps forward, not only for your own personal quality of life, but for humanity as a whole.

WHAT IS PAIN... REALLY???

I love to use acronyms, and for me, pain is Peace Acknowledged In Nature. To many who struggle constantly with pain, this may sound ridiculous; but if we look at pain through a different lens, we can see its deeper value as well as a way out of its prison.

Pain is a language our cells use to let us know they need something. It is like a baby crying. You wouldn't ignore or drug a crying baby; you would give it what it needs to be safe and feel loved. From this perspective, our cells need something other than what we are giving them (because right now, most of us are beating them up).

Think of the messages you send yourself and your cells. If you are in pain, you may hate your body. Likewise, you may resent its limitations, or you may treat it with substances in an attempt to ignore it. You may even give up on it and choose a life of immobility and depression. This is not uncommon in today's world . . . and it's not your fault.

What your cells are really saying to you is that they need space. Without that, they are hungry and dirty. Think of how you feel when you are hungry and dirty yet expected to continue to work hard. It doesn't feel very good. In fact, it can be downright painful.

When your cells have optimal space, they enjoy unlimited flow of blood, oxygen, and all the other nutrients they require. The body supplies what it needs to thrive; it just has to be sure that everything gets where it's going.

A cell without optimal space has less surface area for the transfer of food and the removal of waste. It becomes exhausted and congested. It then sends the brain a message (pain) to let it know its needs aren't being met. If the message is ignored or masked, it will get a little louder. A crying baby left alone eventually starts to scream.

To begin healing, we must understand what the message of pain is saying. Then we must change how we deal with it. It is important to remember that pain is essential to our survival. It provides crucial information about our internal state. Without it, we would remain stuck in self-destructive habits.

Pain is part of the human condition and we need to embrace it. We need to change from bully to friend. Instead of beating up our already exhausted and congested cells with negative attitudes and toxic substances, we need to give them love and proper nutrition. This may sound crazy if you are suffering, but your cells will respond quickly to internal dialogue and right action.

So what is your best course of action when you are living with chronic pain?

In my own journey, I began as most of us do — young and brave, feeling completely in control of my body. I was agile and could perform most athletic feats with ease. I loved the way my body responded to physical challenges and felt invincible.

Then came puberty. Seemingly overnight, I gained twenty pounds, developed hips and breasts, and had to learn to manage the added weight and pressure. I hated it. That started me on a negative course of action, beginning with my internal dialogue: always looking to what was lost and fearing the future. Even the contraption of my first bra with its band of tension around my chest forced physical reactions, with breathing becoming shallow and rapid.

Eckhart Tolle, in The Power of Now, shares that breathing diaphragmatically induces a state of relaxation whereas breathing with the upper chest generates a frequency of stress. It becomes a vicious cycle — pain, fear, and stress cause us to reactively hold the breath, which limits oxygen, thus causing more pain, fear, and stress.

I saw this in myself. As I moved into adulthood, to cope with my discomfort on various levels, I developed an eating disorder, used alcohol to numb myself, worked out in extremely forceful ways, and relentlessly criticized my body. I ended up in many unhealthy relationships, professional and personal. And inevitably, my cells revolted.

When I turned thirty, I made my first decision to move forward to be free again: lose the drinking, which eliminated the guilt and shame of hangovers. A clear mind and body sparked new energy and, even more importantly, compassion for myself though the reflection on my past choices, many bad ones, bred anxiety attacks.

One night, I had a severe attack. I couldn't breathe. I thought I was going to die. Intuitively, I dove my hand into my belly. A gasp of built up tension exploded from me.

Everything that was to come was born in that moment. I encountered pain, but the pain brought me back to reality. With the pressure of my fingers on my abdomen I also noticed something interesting: I was marbled with scar tissue even though I had never had an injury or surgery there. A further awareness dawned. With the gasp of relief, I had recognized my failure to breathe properly and the resultant collapse of my ribcage into my core.

After the attack, I began to study and practice Yoga (another forward-moving habit). That, coincidentally, enabled me to appreciate from experience that most of us habitually vacillate between holding the breath and taking shallow breaths. We had lost our connection with the diaphragm, and our bodies were starving for oxygen.

I have an addictive nature, and this active healing became my new addiction — one with only positive side effects. My mental anguish was dissipating, my self-loathing was supplanted by hope and excitement, and my chronic pain was lessening. Every day since then, I have pursued the process faithfully and thankfully, and I continue to experience the benefits twenty years later.

Tapping into my body with love, compassion, pressure, and breath, I have made pain my friend. It has brought peace to my soul, love to my heart, and freedom to my body. Paradoxically, the key to relief from suffering has proven to be PAIN: Peace Acknowledged In Nature!

Pain, fear, and stress all cause an automatic response in the body. Notice for yourself what happens in the face of any one of these triggers: you reactively hold your breath. For instance, public speaking may make your breathing shallow and rapid, and the volume of your voice decreases until you are frozen. (If this happens to you, take a moment to consciously exhale, push out the stress, reclaim control of the diaphragm, and release the negative energy. You can practice this in private until your exhalation becomes the automatic response to a trigger.)

Another problem that awakened me to the power of conscious exhalation was blushing. It is not uncommon to have low self-esteem and insecurity; as such, frequently blushing, or going red in the face, is a very public way to show self- consciousness. The same conscious breathing exhalation as noted above can work for this, too.

It is empowering to exercise that kind of control over your own physiology. You may still blush if caught off guard or if you say something bolder than perhaps appropriate, but have faith in your ability to get on top of it before it spins into chaos. You can also just laugh about it and not judge yourself so harshly.

We should always bear in mind that pain, fear, stress, and breath restriction work together to reinforce each other.

Let's look at another common scenario. A pain surfaces in your body seemingly out of nowhere. Maybe it is in your gut. For most of us, thoughts of disease and potential death creep to mind as we search for reasons for the discomfort. You make an appointment with a specialist, but you have to wait months for the day to arrive.

Now the pain/fear cycle begins. The reaction to the pain alone causes you to hold the breath. However, the underlying reason for the pain is the cells' lack of blood and oxygen. As you wait for your appointment, your fears grow in anticipation of the diagnosis. This constricts the diaphragm even more, further limiting your oxygen intake, causing more pain, which creates more fear, . . . and so on.

There is good news though. All this is tied to the fascia.

In traditional medical terms, fascia is the equivalent on the inside of the body to the skin on the outside – it ties everything together. But contemporary medical research has focused increasingly on the implications of this and discovered a fascinating wealth of influences extending from the individual cells to the very nature of consciousness.

I personally like to think of the fascia as a fabric, like a sheet. Among other things, it absorbs whatever non-solid medium into which it is immersed. A white sheet will quickly soak up a red wine spill. The wine doesn't alter the shape of the fabric, but it changes the color as well as the smell, and, if you put your tongue to it, the taste. Another type of liquid might even change the texture.

You could also think of a honeycomb. The fascia is the cell walls; the cells and all the life inside them is the honey. Another good analogy is the pixels in a television. The picture comes through the holes (the cells), but without the structure around them (the fascia) the holes don't exist; therefore, no picture would be possible.

What is it that allows the color, smell, taste, and texture to change? It is the space between the fibers of the fabric. Something really dense, like a glass, doesn't absorb: it contains.

The fascia is a container that absorbs. Your environment and all it encompasses — the air you breathe, the water you drink, the food you eat, the relationships you have, the mindset you own, the information you learn — gets stored in this fabric somewhere in your body. Over time, this turns that fresh white sheet into a dirty, smelly, wrinkled, even ripped one.

The good news is that you can wash it, iron it, make it smell clean and fresh, and even mend those tears, *no matter when you start your repairs.*

Not long ago I had the pleasure of meeting a mother and daughter at one of the intensive classes that my nephew and I teach. These classes are a combination of Fluid Isometrics and Block Therapy. The daughter was around my age; her mother, Mabel, was 86 years old. Neither of them had done Block Therapy previously.

Mabel, the mother, was a little anxious at first. She shared that she had struggled with breathing since the age of three, when she had experienced a trauma that left her with Post Traumatic Stress Disorder. She also had pain in her left gluteal and leg — a typical sciatic issue — and problems with digestion and elimination. Also, although lean in build, she was frustrated with her ballooning belly.

A quick note here. People ask me all the time, "Am I too old to start this practice?" Many seniors do Block Therapy, but rarely does someone start at 86. She proved easy to teach and help heal as she truly trusted the process. She and her daughter attended classes monthly, and in between, blocked daily.

Some people are perhaps skeptical of Fluid Isometrics and the science behind the practice. These repair sessions have relevant traditional medical applications as well. About six months into the process, Mabel sent me an email sharing what had happened at her ophthalmology appointment. She told me that the doctor was surprised that her glaucoma test's pressure reading had dropped from 15 and 16 at her last appointment to 9 and 10 at this one. He said he didn't know what she was doing as this never happens, but whatever it was, she should keep doing it! She also mentioned that she had found some old clothes that hadn't fit her for years that she can now wear without discomfort. She ended the email by saying that she feels like she is on the right path and getting healthier every day!

When you open the channels for flow in your fascia and feed oxygen to your cells more completely, things improve: your body moves with greater ease, your systems work with greater efficiency, you have greater control of your emotional responses, and your mind is more clear . . . to name but a few of the benefits.

Our bodies have been in a state of hibernation. It's time to wake them. Winter is over and a new cycle is beginning.

In Fluid Isometrics, you get assistance from a trained healer to locate the multiple sources of your adhesions and pain. Block Therapy teaches you how to be your own pain seeker and healer. In both cases, you focus your attention on what most needs it, connect to the pain, acknowledge it, and give it what it requires. You also wind up discovering pain you didn't know you had. If you dive deep enough into the body, you find that pain is everywhere because no cell is exactly where it should be. Adhesions develop to provide some stability, but they also block blood and oxygen. It seems like you can't win, but you can! Pain is your roadmap.

END YOUR CHRONIC PAIN

A lmost all of us have some amount of chronic pain. Chronic and acute pains are two very different animals. Acute pain occurs in the moment, from a force that enters the body and the resultant damage to the area. It isn't difficult to understand why an ankle is sore if it has just been sprained. Chronic pain, on the other hand, surfaces without any immediate event — it comes when your body can no longer adapt.

Humans are incredibly adaptable creatures. If your shoulder becomes sore from overuse, you simply change the way you use it and continue your actions. This can go on for years, seemingly without cost . . . until the bill arrives. Suddenly you are playing your sport of choice, or gardening, or simply getting out of bed, and your body begins to scream. This causes confusion as there was no apparent moment that resulted in this condition. Your mind races, thoughts of disease and a life of immobility flood your brain, and fear takes hold. Your breath becomes more shallow, your cells become still more starved, and you are set in a cycle of suffering.

Most of us have had this experience. When it happens, you may seek therapeutic or medical attention. Improvements may be temporary at best, leaving you in a state of diminishing returns. Many choose to accept their condition (because they don't know another way) and go on living in the limited capacity their body allows. This takes away joy and leaves more pain and suffering.

With *chronic pain*, the first thing you need to understand is that your fascia has been protecting your body from the external pressures in life. For example, each adjustment you make to your posture prompts the fascia to realign with your off balance body. It grips and adheres to bone to keep you from tipping over. This is the fascia at work; it does it from head to toe.

Pain and its causes are often in different locations. There are also multiple cause sites for pain that need to be addressed in order to bring balance, harmony, and freedom back to movement. This may sound overwhelming - it's actually simple if you know the path and have the discipline to spend the time.

An advantage of the Block Therapy system as it relates to exercise is the isometric component. This gets really interesting when you start to dive deeper into the practice. The purpose of lying on the block is to restore the space in tissue that has been lost over time. An example is work on the hip flexor, where you are draped over the block, allowing the tool to sink into the front of the pelvis, where compression is extreme.

When you elevate the leg of the hip on which you are lying, you are pulling the fascia that has sunk into the hip joint space through years of unconscious posture, and drawing the cells in the gluteus muscles back into proper alignment. When you isometrically hold the position and use your full diaphragmatic breath to feed the cells, you make gains quickly and safely, acquiring an improved ability for movement and exercise.

Let's look at some examples of chronic pain. Based on my experience working with thousands of patients, I can tell you that no matter what the name given to a condition, the underlying reason for it is that cells are blocked from blood and oxygen flow. The affected tissue manifests symptoms that have a name.

The diaphragm is the most important muscle to exercise (and it's why I start the modality work with this first). It feeds every cell with oxygen. The brain dies if deprived of oxygen for five minutes. Each cell is the same — it needs oxygen to thrive.

The cool part is that when you learn to breathe diaphragmatically, and specifically target the exhalation phase, you learn to do core contractions on a continual basis.

This is the best core workout there is. The diaphragm is a huge muscle; you just don't see it as it is hidden inside. What we don't see we tend to ignore, so many don't even think to exercise this muscle. However, it is the muscle that will change your entire shape. In strengthening it, you align the rib cage, detoxify tissue, tone and strengthen the core, and support posture. You also create peace within, as it assists in moving out trapped emotion. The benefits to making this muscle your focus goes beyond what can be conveyed in words. They are felt immediately and continue with practice.

Here are three common issues beyond those associated with basic breathing.

General Movement

We all know the saying: "An ounce of prevention is worth a pound of cure." Isn't it funny how for us to value something, it often has to be taken away? We take our health for granted. We don't usually think about the body unless it is in pain.

Take your feet. These exceptional instruments carry the weight of your whole body, yet are often jammed into containers that throw off your foundation. A pair of high- heeled shoes forces your feet to carry you while bound in a straight jacket. The consequences are far from elegant.

To live the life we have the potential to live, it requires us to consider every cell. This isn't hard to do; it just has to become a habit. The body knows. You don't need a master's degree in how it works; you just need to provide the basics. The same things that you would give your kids, you should give your cells: love, attention, rest, water, oxygen, nutrition, freedom, safety . . . it's called self-care.

I was really fortunate. While developing Fluid Isometrics, I found a way to strengthen my body without force. When I work on patients, I apply isometric pressure deeply into the fascia with both hands while focusing on my diaphragmatic breath. The breath drives the strength and endurance that enable me to administer balanced, continual, fluid force. Isometrics resistance literally means contraction without changing muscle length, so movement into the patient's body doesn't come from my shoulders, elbows, or hands; it comes from the diaphragm muscle moving up and down in the core, and from core contractions.

I have tested this theory and found it true. My work became my exercise. As the years progressed, I developed this ability to maintain isometric pressure for hours at a time. As the work is driven by the breath, not only are the cells constantly being fed so they don't fatigue, they are also constantly being cleaned. This means no lactic acid buildup; it is removed continually, leaving the body free of stiffness.

We tend to think strength requires big muscles. It does not. What is required is each and every cell working for the body, and constant flow of oxygen and removal of waste. To achieve strength and endurance, we must make feeding the cells optimal amounts of oxygen our primary goal. This is also essential to the prevention of injury and disease.

Where Fluid Isometrics is the strategy, Block Therapy is exercise, meditation, and therapy in one. No matter what draws you initially to this work, it is all three things and one leads to the other. Many start because of pain, and then once the pain is gone, they typically continue with the practice because the benefits are so far- reaching. We never know how good we can feel until we feel it. Such experience teaches us to be proactive with our health as opposed to reactive.

Prevention refers not only to the physical body, but also the emotional and mental bodies. When your diaphragm is strong, you are master of your internal world. Our breath regulates our mood, awareness, and connection to the outer world. A body with a weak diaphragm is like a rudderless boat — at the mercy of waves and wind; it leaves you open and vulnerable to people and events. But, if you are connected to the strength of your breath, you can direct your emotions out, gain some influence over your heart rate and anxiety levels, even control your reactions in the moment. A strong diaphragm puts you in charge of your inner life so you allow what serves you to remain and discard the rest.

Block Therapy also teaches you how to overcome fear. FEAR is False Energy Acting Real. How often are your emotions dominated by fear: of disease, of injury, of aging? When you know how to take care of yourself, you have confidence. This breeds inner peace. Things happen, but with a healthy, spacious system, you heal quickly.

I often read testimonials in my professional network from individuals who fell and thought they were badly hurt, but got on the block and did what they knew how to do. They were blown away by how quickly they recovered. One of my own teachers wrote about a burn she got while reaching into her oven and how fast it healed.

When your system is properly fed and cleaned on a regular basis, it can handle efficient tissue repair.

Stress is a constant. Your physical/emotional/mental being rubs against the world around you, and it is relentless. But we don't have to surrender to outside forces and allow whatever comes into consciousness to affect our internal state. We also don't have to wait until pain demands it to practice self-care. No matter how you feel, improving blood and oxygen flow to cells will make things better. So why procrastinate?

Posture and the Spine

Another chronic problem that people typically associate with aging is posture, but it really starts much earlier than retirement! From the moment you are born, gravity is pulling you down. This keeps you on earth, but it also becomes the engine of your aging.

The body is designed to be healthy and thrive. It has built in mechanisms to preserve homeostasis - the tendency toward a relatively stable equilibrium between interdependent elements, especially as maintained by physiological processes. However, the body also adapts to accommodate constant influences - developing, for instance, a characteristic posture over time according to how it is used.

Think of a building with a weak foundation. The first house I ever owned was built in the forties on a riverbank. By the time I purchased it, the original structure had two additions. But the foundation wasn't solid. When you walked from one room to another, you would be going either up or downhill depending on your direction. Eventually, this caused greater problems that were costly and time consuming all because the foundation was weak.

We have foundations built into the body to keep us upright and aligned. But as with anything, if you don't take care of them they begin to decline. Unfortunately, we aren't taught about the importance of proper posture and diaphragmatic breathing.

As kids, we were told to sit up straight. There is more to this than we realize, as posture is the physical representation of the fascia. When imbalance and asymmetry are present, blood and oxygen flow are blocked. As a result, cells don't receive the nutrients they need, and are not kept properly clean, which results in an acidic environment ripe for disease.

I have an ability to see patterns, particularly in posture. Something that disturbs me deeply is the posture of today's youth. Young people are in turmoil. Their bodies in particular reveal one of the negative effects of technology. Growing up in front of computer screens, tablets, and phones is proving catastrophic - they are aging rapidly and have the symptoms to show it.

As I had been working with the fascia for tens of thousands of hours, on patients and myself, I had found a way to move my hands through the layers and untie the seams that time had woven into our bodies. As we age, we compress - we get shorter and wider. Compression is a constant, as gravity is continually pulling us down. Adhesions develop and seal us in unhealthy postures; Fluid Isometrics releases these unnatural bonds.

Better yet, I can teach this technique to others. In my yoga studies, I learned that everyone is born into this lifetime with a signature posture and that it is a goal of each lifetime to break through this hereditary manipulation of one's body. Do you have to accept that just because bunions run in the family that you are destined to get one?

This makes sense to me because through breath we can change our entire physiology. For the first nine months of your existence, you live off your mother's body, energy, and rhythms. You develop in sync with her until you are born and have additional energies to confront and integrate. Many of your response patterns are already programmed into your fascia. Your breath is the mechanism whereby you unconsciously respond to external stimuli, so many of your mother's ingrained responses will also be yours. If mom was prone to anxiety, you likely will be, too. Breath is driven by a muscle, and this gives you your starting point.

One of the central components to posture is literally in the center, at the bottom of your rib cage. The diaphragm is a plate that moves up and down in the core of the body, driving the influx and outflow of air through the lungs. Emotionally, the left (female) side of the body is connected to sadness, the right (male) side to anger.

To see how these factors can create affliction, consider this scenario. A woman is married to a man with anger issues. He has a short fuse and living with him is intense. The woman unconsciously protects herself by contracting her diaphragm to keep her vulnerable insides safe. Every time he comes home, speaks, yells, she does this contraction as pain, fear, and stress cause her to hold her breath.

At the same time she constricts her left side (her heart side) to stop the flow of tears because she knows it will incite more anger in her spouse. If these stimuli are constant over years, eventually that part of her diaphragm will freeze, shifting the alignment of her core.

When one side of the core collapses, the hip joints rotate and the legs adapt to reestablish balance in the body. The leg on the longer side will splay farther from midline; it will also rotate outward and the ankle will have to collapse (pronate) to manage this shift in alignment.

From there, the ball of the foot splays and the resultant mechanics of the woman's gait are skewed. Every step she takes furthers a shifting of fascia in and between the bones of her feet. This puts excessive pressure on the first metatarsal joint and chronic inflammation develops. A bunion forms from the build up of frozen inflammation, originally sent to deliver healing proteins to the damaged area. If the woman doesn't correct the cause of her condition, over time the damage and inflammation increase and the bunion grows.

This is an example of how the signature posture (or, more specifically, the signature breath) affects the physical alignment of the fascia, and of how time manipulates and changes the body. Fortunately, what has been done can be undone without surgery as can other skeletal dysfunctions.

Osteoarthritis is a specific bone-related condition in which the cartilage between the joints wears, causing inflammation and eventual degeneration. This condition is directly attributable to posture. It can occur in any joint in the body and sometimes presents in multiple joints.

Consider a typical approach to an arthritic knee. If pain develops in the knee, a common response is to take anti-inflammatories and for a while it works. The problem is that inflammation is the increased blood flow the body sends to the site to heal it.

So, the area is damaged, and the inflammation that would be used to rebuild tissue is now being forced to stop. The wear and tear continues. The body is adaptable and can handle a lot, but there will always come a point where there is no room left for error. This is when the pain can no longer be controlled. The cartilage has worn away much more than it had at the beginning. Limping may be constant, adding that much more stress to the entire body, and most activity will be put on hold until that inevitable knee replacement.

A different approach at the start would have resulted in a dramatically different outcome. With Block Therapy, the approach is to release the adhesions in the fascia that are blocking blood and oxygen flow. This supports the body's inflammatory response and assists with the natural healing process. Full conscious breathing promotes circulation and oxygenation as well as detoxification; postural foundation building re-aligns the joints to minimize and prevent wear and tear on the cartilage.

There's another example of posture-related issues that many people face, some without knowing. In 1990, there was a TV miniseries based on Stephen King's IT (and in 2017 they came out with a movie remake). Comparing the original cast with the later one provides graphic evidence that today's youth are coming from a very different place inside themselves.

They are in turmoil as they are growing up contracted and twisted partly from poor posture due to technology, partly from junk food, partly from today's increased stress levels, and partly from lack of the free play that was normal for people of my generation when we were kids.

I remember climbing trees and hanging off the limbs, running through the neighborhood playing hide and seek, and generally enjoying moving my body as a child loves to do with the freedom to play. But the world has changed. Structured and contained sports have replaced freeform movement as recreation and it has damaged the skeletal infrastructure of many children.

Scoliosis is not just an issue of the spine. It is the result of the limbs torquing on the spine, causing twisting in the core of the body.

The further the fascia is from the diaphragm, the more frozen it is and the stronger its grip on the bones. The fascia in the lower legs, the feet, the forearms, the hands, all have a direct impact on the alignment of the spine. Once you train your eyes to recognize proper alignment in the fascia, it is easy to notice how the winding of this tissue manipulates the entire body.

Very commonly, I see one leg closer to the midline of the body, the other pulling away. This means the body has shifted its center of gravity in order to stay upright. When you examine the tissue in the lower legs in such a case, you find one calf smaller and denser to the touch, while the other has migrated around the shinbone, strongly hooking around the ankle. This causes the ankle joints to collapse (pronation), bringing imbalance to the foundation of the body and affecting everything up the chain.

From this point, if a person plays a sport, there will be repetitive rotation from one direction to the other. Most, if not all, sports bring on or exacerbate this asymmetrical rotation. If your foundation is already imbalanced, it won't be long before a curve in the spine develops. Playing an instrument is similar in effect. I have seen many who play guitar or violin contort their bodies when they practice. There is a shifting that naturally takes place in the body to handle momentary imbalances, but over extended periods this will seal. Our habitual actions all add up to create our body's alignment.

From a conventional medical perspective, there isn't a lot one can do about scoliosis except try to minimize the curve's descent with an uncomfortable brace, and once that no longer works, a dreaded surgery – spinal fusion – which leaves the body extremely limited in its range of motion. This isn't something that any parent or child would want as it is a life changer.

My first patient with scoliosis was a teenage boy. He was extremely twisted and had a lot of pain as well as other issues originating from the compression of his organs. The doctors said he likely wouldn't live past the age of 21. Block Therapy hadn't been developed when we began his sessions; he was receiving weekly Fluid Isometric treatments.

Within a short time, positive changes were happening. He was becoming more mobile, more aligned; he was gaining weight and was getting happier. All the therapists in my clinic who were learning Fluid Isometrics felt excitement about his progress. Seeing this young man's transformation gave us hope that we were doing something of consequence.

It was during this time that Block Therapy began to take shape as a practice to teach others self-care. It was important to give this young man the tools to continue to look after his body on his own. He joined the first Block Therapy Teacher program and learned the skills to manage his healing and continue to improve lifelong.

Long experience has convinced me that compression from negative posture, scar tissue from injury and/or surgery, and unconscious breathing are at the root of all suffering. Seeing what contemporary youth have ahead of them arouses in me an urgency to make this information available to them. Their bodies are older in tissue than those of the older in years. It all comes down to flow to and from cells, and the young are physically denser than any generation before. They will experience pain, disease, and decrepitude at a much earlier age than necessary. To me this is unacceptable because there is a solution for children and adults alike.

The process is simple, but discipline and action are required. Only dedicated daily work can release the grips that have seized the body, re-align the cells, and reduce/eliminate the curve in the spine. Ultimately, unconscious habits need to change and a new awareness of how to use the body must be acquired. This may sound arduous, but it's the way the body is intended to function, so it is the most natural thing to do. You just have to remember how.

I have worked and am working with many teenagers with scoliosis. A common factor in all my cases is that the parent, usually the mother, feels guilty for not having noticed the problem in its early stages. Parents, I assure you: it's not your fault. This is a function of an increasingly callous world. Nobody is given the proper tools to look after the physical container. How to breathe, how to move, how to allow emotions to surface, how to move them out so they don't fester: these are the things they should be teaching in schools. We need to learn how to keep our bodies healthy and strong, and to teach our kids so they can grow up to be healthy adults.

And teenagers need other teenagers to encourage them.

I am very pleased with one of my patients who will be taking a leading stand in the community to get youths on the Block. I started working with her when she was fourteen. Her scoliosis hadn't been noticed earlier because her head sat straight on her shoulders. She had a forty-five degree upper and thirty-five degree lower curve. It was just assumed she had a short torso with long legs. It wasn't until an X-ray showed the deviations in her spine that she was sent to have a brace made.

She was referred to me by a chiropractor and I created a personalized program for her. In three days, her Mom sent me an email, informing me that her daughter's feet had grown by more than a shoe size. Even I was shocked at the rapid change. She continued, and in two short months her height had increased by two and a half inches. She hadn't been able to grow that much in a year, but the work was undoing all her adhesions, which allowed her to own her true stature. Her standing posture completely transformed and the follow up x-ray revealed a significant reduction in the curve.

It's never too late if you have the will and the way. (Fluid Isometrics and Block Therapy are a way!)

Take this example. A few years back, I started working with a man who was headed for a knee replacement. His leg was twisted at the knee joint, his toes pointed out like a duck's foot, and there was a major collapse in his ankle joint. We had some work to do, but he was willing to embrace Block Therapy as a home program as well as see me weekly for three months for treatments (his surgery was scheduled for the end of that time).

When you are dealing with something that has been ongoing for this long (long enough to require a replacement), there is considerable damage that needs to be addressed; it takes time and dedication to see results. It's wonderful when someone can understand this point at the outset because he or she is then open to the fact that change will not happen overnight. Many give up too soon, as impatience gives rise to unrealistic expectations.

With a three-month window, I felt we had a shot at preventing the surgery. And that is exactly what happened. In fewer than three months, he knew he wouldn't require it and cancelled the operation. I saw him two years later for an unrelated injury and he shared that the knee had not bothered him since.

Taking another common source of skeletal chronic back pain, a herniated disc in the low back is another common complaint. This condition can be extremely debilitating and is often accompanied by referred sciatic pain down the legs. Treatments can vary, but typically it is the low back that is targeted. This, however, is simply the focal point of the full body's collapse of posture. Let me explain.

Fascia grips and adheres to bone with a force up to 2000 pounds per square inch — that's slightly less than the weight of a midsize car! The further an area is away from the diaphragm, the more frozen the tissue so the stronger the hold. The lower legs and feet are the coldest parts of the body due to this distance from the core. If a leg is twisted, it affects the alignment of the pelvis. No one's alignment is perfect, but when there are issues in the low back, the lower legs and feet are one of the primary cause sites for the pain.

Low back treatment will provide only temporary relief from pain as gravity will continue to torque and pull the dense frozen fascia in the legs and feet with every step taken. You can see in the posture of someone with back problems that the legs aren't symmetrical and the body is pulled forward. So for instance, if the body is being pulled to the left, the right low back will be stressed; the collapse of the anterior left pelvis squeezes the vertebrae and causes the disc to shoot out in the equal opposite direction (i.e. the right low back).

Treating the cause sites as well as the pain sites are the focus of Block Therapy. To solve a problem we must recognize its source. Any remedial efforts applied to the actual pain site will prove temporarily effective at best as the very act of walking continues to drag on the already weakened area.

A couple of years back, a woman reached out to me after searching on-line for a solution to scoliosis. I immediately connected with her on Skype.

Edna lives in Puerto Rico. I wouldn't be able to work with her with Fluid Isometrics as I had with my knee patient, so I guided her through Block Therapy. From our conversation, I had no doubt she was invested in doing the work as she had struggled most of her life. On top of the scoliosis, she had herniated discs, spondylolisthesis, chronic back pain . . . and more.

After two weeks, this incredible soul reached out and told me that her menopausal symptoms were gone. She continued her Block Therapy and a short time after that, her scoliosis had improved immensely, her body was re-aligning, and her pain was diminishing. Wanting to share the benefits with as many people as possible, she completed my teacher training program, translated my Block Therapy University courses into Spanish, and opened doors to that many more souls.

Headaches and/or migraines

Another common chronic pain issue is headaches and/or migraines. As with anything else in the body, the pain site and cause site are at different locations. The ribcage is the foundation of the head and neck. If the ribcage has collapsed into the core (and for most people it has), it will pull the head forward out of alignment, and depending on which side of the body is dominant, as well other factors like past injury and surgery, the head will also tilt to one side.

The carotid arteries are positioned at the front of the neck and run behind the clavicle (collar bone). When the head is pulled forward, these bones act like a dam to the flow of blood and oxygen. This is what causes pain, so to attend to the head and neck, or simply provide painkillers, won't get at the root of the problem.

No matter what brought on the issue in the first place (car accident, fall, sitting in front of the computer all day . . .), what needs to happen is for flow to be restored to the head and neck. Oxygen needs to be driven there and upper body alignment needs to be improved and strengthened. This starts with work on the core and ribcage - another benefit, as the pain site doesn't have to be addressed immediately. For some, when the pain is present, even a small amount of pressure on the area can be unbearable. This way, the body can begin healing a comfortable distance from the pain as work proceeds gradually toward the trouble zone.

I cannot stress it enough: all chronic pain issues originate at cause sites a distance from the pain. Effective treatment means approaching the body holistically. Fascia connects you from head to toe; everything affects everything else. The Block Therapy system always considers the entire body and its alignment when seeking a solution to a problem.

I have been working with a friend of mine for years. She has suffered terribly from migraines and general body pain, and when she first came to me, I started working on her obvious cause sites of her rib cage and core. I could see she wasn't breathing effectively so I knew we had to strengthen this to support proper oxygenation to her head/ brain. There were immediate improvements, but she was facing significant challenges.

As a young girl, she was a horseback rider. The resultant posture alone had an impact on her overall alignment and well-being, but in addition, she underwent a lot of trauma to her system trying to get pregnant. She was successful and has two amazing and healthy boys to show for it, but it took a toll on her body. She was struggling daily with pain, using medication to get by.

During the years I worked on her, her condition was constantly improving; her need for medication was diminishing, the intensity and frequency of her migraines were lessening. Her life overall was looking up. But it was when I started to focus on her lower legs, specifically the right lower leg, that a new change took place.

One day she came for a treatment and I concentrated on her lower legs. As we unwound the fascia from her right shin, she suddenly looked smaller and her gait completely transformed. She was walking with grace and ease and her body had a symmetry and balance to it that I hadn't seen previously. It was as if an anchor had been unchained from her; she moved with a lightness that brought a huge smile to her face. She felt the immediate release and saw the change to her size and shape and delighted in them. To this day she continues to work on herself and knows what cause sites she needs to focus to keep advancing.

As I and the many others who have learned how to undo the damage that has led to chronic pain have discovered, it takes time. Know the rewards are assured. Proof and encouragement come regularly as there are always immediate improvements. The changes and relief affirm that we are not merely giving ourselves temporary relief, but fashioning bodies that will be able to respond effectively to future challenges.

PREVENT YOUR ACUTE INJURY

Acute injury is straightforward; if you bang against something, it hurts. There is no denying pain in your ankle when it is sprained, or your hip if you fall on your side. And what is your immediate response to hurting something? You apply pressure or rub it.

Pressure overrides pain. Pressure fibers are bigger than pain fibers. So if something hurts and you rub it, the pressure fibers obstruct the pain signals. This is the science behind a TENS machine, which stimulates pressure fibers around a painful site.

Although ideas about icing are slowly changing, when I was in university to become an Athletic Therapist, we learned the RICE principle - Rest, Ice, Compression, and Elevation. This combined therapy is to be maintained for the first 48-72 hours after an injury to control and limit inflammation. Even thirty years ago, this didn't make sense to me. Why would our body be designed to respond immediately with inflammation if that is not appropriate?

I have experimented over the years with various supportive techniques and learned a different approach that decreases healing time. Rather than stop the body's natural response, we need to encourage and support it.

The traditional belief is that, if an injury occurs, unless right action is taken, inflammation can get "backed up" and cause more tissue damage. This is the reason we are taught to limit inflammation. However, if we knew how to promote flow and not allow the area to become congested, then that inflammation would rebuild the damaged cells and tissue - and it would do so at a much faster rate.

It's like baking a cake. If you mix flour, eggs, sugar, and oil together, you have batter. The raw materials for the cake are in the batter. If you put that bowl of batter into the freezer, you have frozen batter. If you put it into the oven, you bake a cake. It is the heat that causes the batter to transform into something other than its contents.

When you become injured, the inflammation sent is filled with whatever raw materials your body needs to repair whatever is damaged. The body is ingenious in its design and it knows what it requires to heal. With injury, there are multiple cells that need repair - they may be muscle, tendon, blood vessels, nerve fiber, fat, ligaments . . . many cells get damaged when a force enters the body. To support healing, we must ensure optimal blood flow. If we do this, the body takes care of the rest.

This brings us back to the basics: breath and posture. The best way to ensure you are doing what you need to do to heal as efficiently as possible is to promote optimal oxygenation and removal of waste. The breath drives healing by pumping blood to all the cells. Only the diaphragmatic breath has the power to reach every cell in the body.

Equally important is efficient removal of waste. When a blow impacts your system, there is debris that needs to be taken away from the site of injury and eliminated from the body. Imagine a collision or pile up on the highway. Broken glass, fenders, tires . . . a lot of debris to remove before traffic flow can resume. The same is true in the body after an injury. This is what the full conscious exhalation does.

Apart from working on myself, I tested this theory on my mother. I was working in a clinic at the time and she called me one day from the golf course. She had just hurt her ankle and it sounded pretty bad. I told her to come and see me immediately.

My initial assessment told me she likely had a pretty severe second degree sprain to the lateral ligaments in the ankle, which is very common but also very painful. My training would have had me elevate the ankle and wrap it in ice to provide pressure and reduce inflammation. However, I had something else in mind.

I had hurt myself often enough and always applied my understanding to my own injuries, moving past the pain rapidly. This being my mom, I figured testing my theory on her would be safe enough as she would never let me do something to her that didn't feel right. I got her comfortable on the exam table and slowly started applying direct pressure to the injury.

Initially, she was afraid of the pressure and would pull away; however, we were in no rush, and I knew that if she could settle into her breath and allow me to do my thing, she would calm down. It took only a moment; soon, the pressure was starting to feel good to her. I started with a very light touch, then gradually began applying more. Change was positive; the swelling was quickly moving away from her ankle and her mood was lightening.

After the session, I had her get up to walk. At first she was tentative about putting weight on the foot. I took her hand and stood beside her so she would feel safe and supported. I also showed her how to connect her breath to the painful action so she could breathe the damage out of the area and replace it with healing proteins, oxygen, and minerals for repair.

She walked out of the clinic much better than when she entered; I knew, however, that as soon as she rested, inflammation would again fill the injured space as that is what the body does to heal. With this swelling comes pain, so to make sure she understood the process, I told her what to expect, and how to manage until the next morning, when I would come to see her at her house. Her self-care included heating the area with a hot pack or taking a bath, moving the ankle in circles and even putting weight on it as her breath allowed, and elevating it to keep the inflammation circulating. (Note: inflammation contains all the nutrients required for healing and rebuilding tissue, but if it becomes stagnant, it creates more problems. Keeping the flow moving is the key to using inflammation to your advantage.)

The next morning, I went to see her and she shared that during the evening the pain had been pretty bad, as I had expected. It was a serious sprain, so whatever pain had entered her body had to come out. In essence, she needed to experience it again as it left. Also, when she took her first step that morning, of course there was a lot of buildup of inflammation that had occurred during sleep, so the ankle felt thick and stiff.

I started working on it right away. She definitely wasn't afraid of the pressure anymore. After the session ended, she stood and walked. It was almost as though there was nothing wrong. She said it felt 70% better that day and it only progressed quickly from there.

A few years later, I encountered a similar acute injury. I was deep into developing Fluid Isometrics when one of my therapists brought me a patient, John, who had fractured his fourth metatarsal bone (one of the long bones in his foot) six days before. He was a provincial rugby player and had Nationals in three weeks. His doctor told him to not weigh the bear for four weeks.

This was exciting as I had yet to work on a bone fracture. I already fully believed that fascia integrated every cell in the body, so why should a bone be different from soft tissue? I started with the basics, knowing that what was needed was proper breath and flow. I began working in his core and ribcage and taught him how to breathe diaphragmatically, then proceeded down the leg, opening all the main channels, until I reached his foot.

Once there, I knew that if I gave him the power to move into the pain that he would feel in control. This would remove his fear of pain rather than if I merely moved his injured limb. As he was lying on his back, I placed my hand on the bottom of his foot and asked him to push into my hand, applying his breath as he did so.

This is crucial when working with people in pain: give them control and they overcome their fear. He started putting pressure into my hand, lightly at first, but it wasn't long before he was pushing beyond what I could counter with my hand strength. At that point I had him stand up and repeat the exercise, this time with his foot moving into the floor. By the end of the session, he could push off with the foot and consciously walk without limping. I gave him some homework to do and had him return the next day.

In total, I worked on him four times between day six and two weeks post injury. He played Nationals the next week, with minimal pain. This was momentous for me; he was the first person I treated for bone fracture.

But the next was soon to follow. A young man from New York reached out to me after seeing John's video on social media. He was a soccer player and had fractured his 5th metatarsal (an injury known as a Jones Fracture). This break is considered slow to heal; often, a metal rod is put into the bone to stabilize the fracture. He needed to get his foot rehabbed quickly as he was about to leave for training in Croatia and his injury was going to set him back.

I agreed to work on him for a week. He arrived in Winnipeg three weeks post injury, wearing a boot and walking with a limp.

I was confident of success, but after the first treatment, even I was blown away by his progress. It was comical because he had only brought one shoe. He had been wearing a boot on his fractured foot for three weeks; it didn't occur to him or his mother to bring the corresponding shoe. After the first day, he was walking with little pain and doing sport specific exercise as though nothing had happened. He had to go to a nearby mall that day to buy a new pair of shoes.

I have had countless such experiences with acute injury and am happy to say that my community has also brought about amazing healings from acute injury by using the block and breath to promote flow as well as utilize the body's innate intelligence. Fear of pain is the only limiting factor. Learning to embrace the body's natural ability to heal in the moment is the most efficient way to repair what is damaged and to prevent chronic issues that result from compensating for injury.

Many acute injuries are simply the result of bad habits, so we should take the time to consider some preventive practices. There are many forms of exercise, and I have tried lots of them. What I have come to understand is that, for the most part, exercise might make you fit, but that doesn't mean it's good for your body.

=Compression is the root of pain, aging and disease. The goal of exercise should be to lengthen and strengthen the body, which would support healthy aging. Working the body with this in mind will assist in countering the constant downward pull of gravity and help to maintain balance and symmetry to ensure optimal circulation.

The combination of oxygenating the fascia to make it physically lighter, and strengthening postural foundations to make the body stronger and more balanced, promotes "effortless effort" - the ultimate path to moving with grace and ease.

People's individual goals with exercise are unique to them; however, the bottom line is that they want to feel and look healthy. Fascia health requires that we support our bodies with flow and freedom of space.

Individual Sports

Though we are free to choose what seems to "work" for us, not all choices are good. Running is another example of counterproductive exercise. Again, keep in mind, nobody is perfectly aligned. Over time, the diaphragm muscle weakens from lazy breathing habits and the ribcage collapses into the core. The weight of the ribcage, head, arms, and hands exerts considerable pressure on the abdomen, challenging the internal organs. Add to this the repetitive pressure of pounding feet on pavement. It is not uncommon to hear of marathon runners who collapse and die at an early age.

Then there is the effect on the joints. Running increases wear and tear, leading to inflammation, pain and eventual arthritis. The inflammation is sent initially to rebuild the area, yet as people don't understand what's happening, they take anti- inflammatories to numb the pain so they can continue to exercise. This adds insult to injury. Pain is a critical message and deserves our respect.

From the perspective of symmetry, tennis is one sport that has sent me a significant number of patients. This sport has the size and weight of the racquet in addition to the force of the ball reverberating through it. The continual pounding, reaching, and follow through from the swing creates a huge imbalance in the size of the arms, particularly forearms.

As soon as the body shifts to handle these repetitive forces, it re-aligns to counter the pull and keep itself upright. This constant adaptation slowly winds it down, taking away space required for the adjustment, until the body hits a proverbial wall causing it to express its pain chronically and loudly.

Pick any sport and you will find that it presents challenges of asymmetry (tennis, volleyball, golf), compression (running, cycling, rowing), or both.

Weightlifting and Bodybuilding

I remember a time in my late teens at the beginning of my university career when I reached an impasse. Having just graduated from a private girls' school, where I excelled in both sports and academics, I suddenly found myself incredibly unhappy with my body. I wanted to be thin, so I began obsessively working out. This didn't achieve the desired result - I kept getting bigger the harder I trained. At one point, when I was doing a hundred push-ups a day, my mother actually said to me, "Your head looks too small for your shoulders".

I was totally deflated. Every night in my bedroom I did those push-ups. I believed that the more muscle mass I accumulated, the higher my metabolism would be and the thinner/smaller I would get. Yet all my hard work had accomplished the exact opposite. I had wanted to be a ballerina, but I looked like a football player.

The workouts made me strong, but also thick and round. Instead of treating my body with care and consideration, I was using force. The repetitive contractions of weight lifting and calisthenics created compression in some areas and ballooning in others rather than lengthening and strengthening tissue in proper alignment.

The Block Therapy system is designed to restore the space that time (and, unconsciously, you) has diminished, fill it with optimal amounts of oxygen, and maintain it by establishing proper postural foundations. This practice took me far from the thick, dense mass my body had become. It took me to a place of health, unprecedented vigor, and control over my reactive emotional being. It took me to where I trust myself and this is the greatest blessing of all. You can achieve this same freedom.

Block Therapy is designed for this purpose. The diaphragm is made to pull oxygen in and eliminate waste. However, in most of us, and especially the young, it is locked far away from conscious awareness, frozen and immobile. It takes some effort to connect with it, but once you do, everything changes.

The body's pressure fibers are larger than its pain fibers. Lying on the Block while connecting to the diaphragm transforms the sensation of pain to one of pressure, or good pain as many call it. Feeling the inner shifts enables you to trust the process and know the work is helping.

The procedure is also easy. No skill is required, just following directions. You literally lie on the tool, move into the pain as instructed, using your breath as your guide, and let the process happen. From there, the foundation work is integrated. Learning how to sit, stand, and move correctly is a necessary component for change, but again, it isn't hard to do; it's simply in the doing that the changes occur.

If you want to build your body, think long-term. If you care about your body now, you will care in twenty, forty, even sixty years. Do today what will make your tomorrows vigorous and active. Block Therapy will teach you a healthy approach to developing a body that will serve you well your whole life long.

The body is the temple of the soul. Proper care of this gift is the highest tribute we can pay to ourselves and the world around us. When you take the time to reflect on how truly remarkable the body is, it becomes easier for you to give it the attention and love it deserves.

My goal was to be lean. Unfortunately, the more I worked out, the bulkier I became. As an Athletic Therapist, I had learned what I needed to do to get the fit body I wanted, yet my attempts always ended up with me injured and bigger than before I began the work.

Over time I have learned that traditional body building practice isn't healthy. For individuals striving to become as big as they can, there is a component of force that is detrimental to cells. There can be only so much expansion before internal pressure becomes excessive. As well, supplements and other unnatural means of generating mass cause cells to balloon beyond a healthy size. Initially this may have the desired effect, but long term the cells become weak and toxic, leading to serious health problems.

A better approach to building a healthy, fit body would be to sculpt the form to its own natural size and proportion. Instead of spending time in the gym, repeatedly going through a series of reps to make an area bigger, concentrate on releasing areas blocked from blood and oxygen flow, then strengthening proper alignment through isometric resistance. Once the body has strong and aligned foundations, more traditional training can then add mass in a healthy way.

Let's compare these two approaches and see results.

Say you wanted to increase the diameter of your chest. Traditionally, you would go to the gym and do exercises to build it, using free weights or machines like the Pec Deck that target this muscle group. Whatever your method, you repeatedly contract the muscles in an attempt to make them stronger and harder. So, you may ask, what's the problem?

First, anyone beginning a workout program starts with bad alignment - none of us are properly aligned. Strengthening an unbalanced body creates a more unbalanced body, which in turn places greater stress on everything: organs, joints, muscles, ligaments, tendons . . .

Also, the repetitive contraction generates tension in the structures underneath the targeted area. Under the pectoral muscles is the rib cage, which houses the heart and lungs. This protective armor is super strong, in part from its flexibility. Continual repetitive contractions of the pectoralis muscles will cause them to shorten, compressing the rib cage, taking away space from the heart and lungs. This problem isn't immediately evident, but develops over time into serious health issues.

I have seen many bodybuilders with stretch marks in the anterior part of the shoulder, which is a sign that their tissue is ballooning past a healthy level. Stretch marks are scar tissue, and scar tissue blocks blood and oxygen flow to cells. This leaves them starved for nutrients, acidic from toxicity, and ripe for injury and disease. The movements create a tearing in the tissue, causing the body to rebuild. If this is done repeatedly, the muscles become bigger and denser.

But here is the problem: the dense muscles are partly that way because they have shortened; they become shorter and thicker. The shortening shifts the alignment of the body, pulling it forward and accelerating aging. The density also takes away the space between the cells, compromising the flow to and from the area. As we have already discussed, for optimal health, cells need space for the blood flow that feeds and cleans them.

Another drawback of weight lifting is the starting position. Nobody is perfectly aligned. When you strengthen through weight training, you are actively forcing your body further out of alignment. This happens all the time. A person wants to rehabilitate an area and is given strengthening exercises. If the body isn't properly supported in the beginning, the exercises only add stress to the joints.

I cannot repeat it often enough: for cells to be healthy, they need proper flow. Making tissue dense impairs flow to cells causing them to age more rapidly. Although you may feel yourself getting stronger initially with body building exercise, it won't be long before you begin to suffer the negative side effects of injury and muscle imbalance.

Conversely, if you first release the tissue that has become blocked in the ribcage, you begin to awaken and integrate cells, thereby improving flow. This gives you more cells to work with and expand through your exercise, and it lifts the rib cage up and out of the abdomen, freeing the diaphragm muscle (this is also the fastest way to an hourglass figure and strong, healthy abdominal muscles). This approach changes everything, as properly oxygenating your cells is the safest way to increase your strength.

Here is another way to think about flow and oxygen as the fuel for our health. Adenosine triphosphate, or ATP, is a complex organic chemical that uses oxygen and provides energy to drive many processes in living cells, e.g. muscle contraction, nerve impulse propagation, and chemical synthesis (*Purinergic Signal).*

ATP is the engine; oxygen is the fuel. It follows that connecting to your full diaphragmatic breath is the most efficient way to strengthen not only your muscle cells, but all of your cells. Your diaphragm muscle should be the focus of every single workout - not other muscles. Your core connection to this powerful motor will enable you to perform feats of endurance and strength . . . without succumbing to exhaustion.

Try this as a healthier way to strengthen your engine with weights.

If you have free weights, grab two of equal weight, enough that you can lift safely but with some resistance. If you don't have weights, you can grab two cans of equal weight to do this drill. Now sit in a chair and do several bicep curls. Notice any tensions; notice any asymmetries in the way your hands hold the weights. Notice which arm tires faster; notice if you are more collapsed on one side of your rib cage.

Once you have observed yourself and taken note, you are ready to connect to your power posture. Put the weights down and sit with your feet planted firmly on the floor. Slide forward until half your thighs are off the chair. Have your knees bent at ninety degrees and bring them together. Now contract your anus and feel your body shift back. Exhale fully, from your belly. Place your hands on your abdomen as you exhale; feel your belly get smaller. The anal contraction connects you to your root.

Contract with the exhale, then relax as you inhale. Repeat this ten times to own your new alignment.

Now grab the weights again, resume the posture, and when you feel grounded, do your bicep curls, exhaling as you lift. Slow the movement down and notice the changes. Has it become easier to lift the same weight? Look at your hands and see if you can make them look the same - you want symmetry. Is your endurance better?

I remember when I was beginning to teach my nephew, Quinn, who was a Physique Bodybuilder, about using his breath and root when working out. He noticed immediately the ease with which he lifted the same weight that had been challenging to his unconscious posture.

It makes sense. In one respect, the body is like a machine: there is absolutely a way it functions best. We all have different potentials for how big our muscles can get and the healthiest way to build them is within the ranges our breath will allow.

Instead of force, use persuasion.

Through decompression and consequent cell regeneration, more cells enter the equation for increasing size. Not only that, decompression takes massive amounts of pressure off the skeleton, making simply being upright less exhausting, thus enhancing your energy reserves.

When you add isometrics, you pull cells back to their rightful positions, lifting out of hibernation. I like to call it "Owning Your New Space".

When you decompress fascia, space that was lost over time is revealed. If you go back to your unconscious posture, you will collapse that space again. But if you own your new alignment with a combination of isometric holds and fascia decompression techniques, it gets cemented in place. From there, you continue to melt and lift, melt and lift, . . . which brings you back in touch with your core, each breath moving out toxins, inflammation, and waste.

The breath will also keep you safe. There is a difference between being fit and being healthy. The goal is to be both, but the healthy should precede fit.

The body wants to be healthy and breath is the key. As long as you can breathe in a relaxed way with any movement, your cells are being fed and waste is being removed. Your breath, and the continual flow of oxygen to all cells, keeps the engine running. When you exercise to the point where you run out of breath or lift an object heavier than you can comfortably breathe, injury and exhaustion occur.

It is a popular misconception that we have to beat ourselves up to get a strong, toned, and fit body. Yes, many want to push their limits and outperform themselves and others, but that doesn't come from a desire to build a healthy body; it comes from a competitive urge. I am all for healthy competition - it helps us to grow. But like building a sound body in a sustainable way, competition should breed improvements in performance without damaging your or someone else's health. When you find a sport you love, part of what you love is how your body feels doing it. When you regularly practice to the point of pain, eventually the fun is gone and your energy goes into managing chronic pain instead of enjoying an activity that made you feel alive.

Team Sports

As the most competitive form of exercise, sports add an extra measure of stress to the aging process. It's interesting that people assume athletes are healthy. Of course they can outperform the average person in many different ways. Though they may be stronger and faster, have greater endurance, and have better reaction times, this doesn't always translate into good health.

A healthy body, from the perspective of the fascia system, needs to be fluid and spacious. It all comes down to flow. One of the problems with many sports is the asymmetrical bias they foster through right or left side dominance and repetitive actions.

Consider tennis, golf, basketball, hockey, football . . . any sport where your dominant side is slinging an object. This action sets your body up for long-term disaster. The more you practice, the more asymmetrical you become. The repetitive twisting action winds the body, causes it to bind and seal over time, limiting its ability to move freely. The younger you start, the more challenged your fascia system will be to preserve balance and symmetry in your cells. For the masses, sports are a stimulating pastime; for the athlete, they drive the body to premature old age.

Think of a right handed high-level volleyball player, maybe one who plays beach volleyball. Most of these players have a wicked spike, and practice relentlessly. However, this abuses the player's "physical container". I can't even guess how many times these players pull the right arm above the head, preparing to deliver a killer blow to the ball. This causes the ribcage to twist to the left on the delivery of the spike. Considered this way, the repetition generates many chronic pain conditions.

If volleyball competitors understood the fascia system, they would practice using the non-dominant side (here, spiking with the left hand) to create balance and reduce blockages from the twisting and unevenness. This would engender healthier rotation in the core, more balance in the mind, and better overall posture. When you practice with both sides equally, you don't bind and seal in one direction. If athletes would make this part of their training, their bodies would be more supple, have better circulation, and exhibit superior adaptability in times of stress.

I put this "balance" theory to the test playing Ping-Pong. Some of you may not call this a sport, but the eye/hand coordination is intense. You can definitely work up a sweat. I played as a kid and got really good at it; then, years later, my husband and I would play in our basement. We were both equally proficient, so we would spice it up by challenging each other to use the less dominant hand.

This was tons of fun. First came the awkwardness of simply trying to hit the ball, but our skills developed quickly, until, before we knew it, we were able to play - although at a beginner's level compared to when we played with our dominant sides. This was remarkable to us both as it wasn't long before our weak sides didn't seem so weak.

But here is where the magic happened.

When we went back to playing with our dominant sides, we both had improved dramatically. It was then that I realized practicing with your non-dominant side in whatever you do will advance your dominant side's skill that much more quickly.

We have been conditioned to follow beliefs that don't support fascia health. The conventional approach to exercise is to force the body to respond. Your cells do not want to be beaten. They are already working hard on your behalf. That doesn't mean we don't need to exercise or train, but there is a way to do this without compromising our fascia. If you want to enjoy your body to its fullest potential as you age, it requires a little understanding and application.

We tend to think of professional athletes as superhuman and, to some extent, they are - for a time. Unfortunately, many wind up with pain and physical challenges that end their careers in their prime, leaving them with chronic issues. Supporting fascia health with balanced training will produce superhumans with lasting power to not only share their athletic prowess, but to enjoy bodies that age with grace and freedom.

TISSUE TEMPERATURE

The hypothalamus acts like a thermostat for the body, keeping its body's temperature at 98.6 degrees Fahrenheit. If a person's body begins to cool, it will shiver to stimulate blood flow, which will help to increase its temperature. If it becomes too hot, it sweats, pulling salt and water to the skin so evaporation can cool it down. There are many complex communications regulated by the hypothalamus in order to maintain this equilibrium.

When we discuss fascia, we are really talking about cellular alignment. When every cell is properly aligned, there is optimal space in the tissue for cellular communications and exchanges. The cell membrane determines what moves in and out, and at what pace. In perfect alignment, there would be ease of flow; whatever the cell required would be delivered immediately and absorbed through the membrane. Similarly, all cellular waste and toxins would be carried away to be excreted from the body. The flow is driven by the diaphragmatic breath and supported by proper cellular alignment, which requires conscious awareness at all times. In such a body, every cell would be at 98.6 degrees Fahrenheit.

Sadly, our actual reality is quite different. We are not a population that has been conscious of our bodies. We have allowed our breath to become weak and our foundations to tip off balance. Returning to the bunion example, it really starts with an unconscious response to negative stimuli — contracting the diaphragm to ward off unpleasant energy. This repetitive contraction winds, becomes dense, and torques the core out of alignment, thereby forcing a shifting of the body to maintain its balance. The fascia builds false walls and false floors to create a superficial foundation. This arises out of the migration of cells and the compression that results as they stack and stick together.

This dense, sticky tissue lacks flow. It is cold and dirty. Space is required for flow, so taking it away slows and eventually stops flow. You may notice this when certain areas of your body feel colder than others. I first observed the phenomenon in my abdomen when coming back from a run. I would be hot and sweaty, yet my belly felt cold to the touch. This was a huge frustration as my belly was the one area I wanted most to change. But remember, compression from unconscious breathing, incorrect posture, and unhealthy thinking created the density and coldness, leaving those cells blocked from life.

To regulate cellular temperature, we need space for flow with all communication and exchanges driven by the conscious breath. Once you understand this, it is simple to apply Block Therapy because the temperature of your tissue will tell you what needs attention.

For example, most people have cold feet. The cells of the feet are the furthest from the engine (the diaphragm) and the most compressed as they are positioned at the base of the body. The entire weight of the body over time adds up to create more and more compression.

Consider this other fact — there are 26 bones in the feet. It is a huge number for such a small area, but indicative of the amount of adapting to uneven surfaces that can take place to keep the body upright and balanced. If we don't pay attention to how the feet should be positioned for correct alignment, over time the continual adaptation torques the legs, twists the pelvis, and compresses the core. The rib cage gets pulled into the core from the blocked and weakened diaphragm, compressing the abdomen and its contents even further, spiraling the body into an aging pattern accepted as normal today. Your goal: heat the feet!

Spelled out like this, the process sounds simple and in fact it is; it just takes desire and a bit of discipline. You can use Block Therapy as a complete and effective system for heating up cold areas. This happens in three stages:

Step One — Creating Space

The act of lying on the tool, the Block Buddy/Baby, creates pressure in the appropriate area. This causes the cell molecules to accelerate, which generates heat, which then in turn melts the fascial adhesions that have glued the cells together out of alignment. Flow resumes, bringing oxygen, healing nutrients and proteins as well and carrying away toxins with waste that have become trapped.

Adhesions develop throughout the fascia, so to ensure that blood reaches all the places it needs to travel, there is a sequence to the positions. Typically we start working in the core and ribcage. The diaphragm is the body's furnace. If there is compression in the ribcage (and I have yet to see someone who hasn't collapsed there at least to some degree), we need to melt the adhesions that are impeding this muscle's ability to move up and down in the core.

For most people, one class is all it takes to bring about a lifting of the ribcage and a deeper and stronger breath. When this area is targeted as a starting point in Block Therapy, the whole body "breathes a sigh of relief" with the increased oxygenation that occurs.

Step Two — Inflating Space

As suggested, breathing from the diaphragm is like turning on the body's furnace. The diaphragm is the engine that drives the plate of muscle up and down in the core, and moves fluids throughout the body, keeping cells fed and clean. Proper exhalation moves waste out of the body and proper inhalation pulls air to the base of the lungs, where optimal absorption into the bloodstream takes place.

When we are working to improve blood and oxygen flow to the extremities, the breath is always the driver of movement. There is a sequence to the placement of the Block Buddy to help blood and oxygen get to the farthest reaches of the body. Working towards the extremities, melting adhesions along the way gradually opens cells that have been blocked in a systematic order depending on the target area.

To reach the feet, we would first connect to the breath in the core, then work through the pelvis, and symmetrically find our way step by step with the block through the hips, thighs, the knees, calves, and finally the feet. Following this path allows the cells to open and the blood and oxygen to melt each layer, in turn, until we arrive at the feet. If any area is missed, the feet don't get the benefit. Following the designated order ensures that you will efficiently open all channels for optimal flow and melting.

Step Three — Maintaining Space

Correct cellular alignment is the goal if we are to maintain optimal space in our tissue for all cells to function with ease. Space means flow, which is required to maintain cellular temperature. Block Therapy establishes and strengthens proper foundations to support the cells and maintain space.

Keeping the body healthy in this fast-paced and unclean world is a challenge we all must face. It can get overwhelmingly complicated when we separate the body into parts. The fascia connects every cell, and for optimal health, it is the cells that we need to understand. Focusing on tissue temperature is a simple way to recognize where time and attention are most needed. Block Therapy provides a straightforward approach to reviving the cold and dirty spots.

To support lower body foundations and maintain optimal space, we strengthen the root. This is a combination of aligning the feet and legs, activating the proper muscles, and concentrating on balance and symmetry. Sixty percent of the body weight should rest on the heels; for most, eighty percent rests on the balls of the feet through leaning forward.

The diaphragm muscle is the foundation of the ribcage and exercising proper diaphragmatic breathing is the way to strengthen this base as well as to keep it open. The heart and lungs should be at the front of the chest, when, in reality, most have collapsed into their cores, pushing these organs to the back of the body. Toxins and waste accumulate as a result, which can lead to breathing issues and add stress to the heart muscle. Strengthening the diaphragm and opening the chest through the work prescribed in Block Therapy will create a strong foundation to support these life-giving organs.

Maintaining space between the cells through conscious awareness of proper alignment is the third and most difficult part of the Block Therapy process. That said, we make it easy with our user-friendly programs and step by step strengthening and alignment training procedures to ensure optimal benefits and outcomes from the work.

THE FOUNDATION OF DISEASE

What happens to the cells in the body when flow is compromised? Let's consider a river by way of analogy.

I have lived on or near a river my entire life. For the last thirteen years, my home has been on the thirteenth floor of a high rise right on a river's edge. This has allowed me to observe the habits of the river through the changing seasons. It is a good metaphor for the human body, which is, after all, a fluid container.

When the river isn't frozen, there is always foam traveling down the center, typically in a wavelike motion. In one particular place not far up river, a tree had fallen with its trunk extending many feet from the bank into the water. As the foam approached this obstacle, it was pulled toward it as though by force of gravity and the pattern appeared spiral in nature.

As it got closer, however, a chaotic pattern replaced the spiral one. I could see the bubbles trapped in a dizzying vortex, continually accumulating more foam. This area of the river became a harbor for the foam to mingle. The only way to free it from this pattern of chaos would be to remove the fallen tree.

How is this relevant to the health of your cells? All cells need flow to be healthy; barricades to flow create opportunity for debris to get trapped. If toxins, waste, by- products of cell function, or even negative emotion get stuck in a holding pattern, they take away the space that oxygen and other required nutrients need to reach and feed the cells.

Along another river analogy, think of an algae-filled area of water that has been stagnant through the hot summer months. The water has a greenish tinge with an unpleasant smell and you aren't likely to want to take a swim in this infected cesspool. This is water with no flow and it obviously isn't a healthy environment.

A diabetic foot that is gangrenous and on the verge of amputation is similar to this standing water as it is an area with compromised flow that is stagnant and unhealthy. Once the flow is blocked completely, cells begin to decay and eventually this will spread as the microorganisms overrun the healthy tissue. Amputation is one solution to save the life of the person, but removing the barricades to flow would save the life of individual cells.

Let's discuss the removal process. This is where it can get a little overwhelming because everywhere, every cell, every inch of the body, is out of alignment. People don't realize the significance of the entire fascia system connecting every single cell.

To get a basic understanding of this interconnectedness, take a towel and lay it flat on the floor so that it is perfectly aligned and smooth. Now, grab the towel at one of the corners and twist. Notice how the entire towel changes as you do this. The corners on the bottom edge get pulled up, and everything is drawn in toward the source of the twisting.

In a parallel treatment modality called Cranial Sacral Therapy, the twisting point is called an energy cyst. An energy cyst is an area in your body that is pulling the life force out of your tissue like a black hole. It draws everything into it, sucking life and health from the body.

This is what happens to any area that has a barricade, or dam, blocking flow. Just as with the tree in the river, energy is drawn toward the density. An energy cyst accumulates mass, debris, toxins and waste, and the bigger it gets, the more powerful its gravity. A bruise on your thigh, for instance, develops scar tissue in that area and acts like the fallen tree, blocking flow and amassing dirt along with debris. This creates chaos in the flow and blocks the rest of the leg from receiving nutrients.

As I have mentioned before, health requires flow. Flow to and from your cells is dependent on three things: no obstructions, an engine, and an aligned container. Let's look at each of these individually to understand how your body is designed to be healthy.

No obstructions

The body is so incredibly adaptable that we don't even recognize when it shifts to accommodate an area of decreased range or one that suddenly feels pain. Think of throwing a ball, swinging a golf club . . . or an action you do on occasion.

There is a "perfect" form to which we all aspire when engaged in an activity or sport. However, since we aren't perfectly aligned, our bodies adapt their movements to create the desired result. If you are a golfer, you may buy the expensive driver, a new set of golf balls that should allow you ten extra yards, or you may pay a golf pro to guide you on your perfect swing. But if your ribs are glued together because you had a trauma there earlier in life, you will have to compensate for your lack of motion in that area to achieve your aim.

These compensations may work short term. But eventually you hit a tipping point where your body is incapable of any further adaptation, where there is no room left to cheat the system. You find yourself unable to enjoy the game because no matter how you shift, your swing feels labored, inflexible, awkward, and doesn't produce the result that once gave you such satisfaction. Your game is compromised. It doesn't matter what equipment you buy to help improve your swing. It's your body that is failing you.

There is a powerful barricade glued to your bones bearing a 2000 pound per square inch force. The fascia exists to protect and teach us, but if we don't respect it and learn from it, it becomes a nagging presence that leads to chronic pain and anxiety.

An engine

When the body is alive, there are countless unconscious functions taking place, and breathing is one of them. The unique thing about breathing is that it can also be conscious. But the moment a person dies, all movements, cell interactions, and chemical processes cease in the body.

We are designed to survive. This means that even if the body does not have what it needs to *thrive*, it will still function, although at a lesser capacity until it wears out. What's really cool, though, is that when we become conscious diaphragmatic breathers, the body begins to thrive. Breathing consciously is like turning on the furnace or internal engine. When used properly, the diaphragm becomes a pump for fluid transport, oxygen delivery, and waste removal. As long as the engine is functioning and strong (which takes conscious awareness), the cells receive what they need to thrive, waste is efficiently removed, and we are able to maintain a clean and healthy environment.

An aligned container

The cells need space for nutrient reception and waste removal. If a body is collapsed from a lifetime of bad posture, riddled with scar tissue from injury or surgery, or corrupted from abuse, there will be areas lacking in that space.

Proper foundation strengthening and alignment of cells is essential if a body is to thrive. Our amazing adaptability enables us to deal with injury as it arises, but if we don't get back to a neutral alignment after we have healed, the weight of the collapsing body gains momentum, causing fatigue and pain.

Unfortunately, this is the state of the majority of people as they age, and now the negative impact of unconscious posture is rearing its ugly head at an increasingly younger age due to the warping elicited by technology.

If these concerns are addressed, the individual will have space for flow, which means the ability to heal quickly after injury, handle life's stresses, and thrive in whatever activities are undertaken. A conscious person who puts time and attention into the fascia system makes the body a healthy container for a long and productive life.

It is when a person isn't aware of what the cells need that disease creeps into their spaces (and it does creep). How often is someone apparently healthy, only to die months later of cancer that has overrun the body? That is the negative side of our adaptability. If we are not conscious of the signals the cells are sending, then eventually they simply shut down and a breeding ground develops for disease. As in the stagnant water filled with algae, bacteria, fungi, and viruses feed on the microorganisms that thrive in these acidic, dirty environments, and make a home, depleting tissue of health and life.

Let's look at some common diseases and see how taking care of your fascia changes their prospects.

DISCOURAGING SPECIFIC DISEASES

In approaching disease and specific treatments, we must consider which perspective works best for us. Conventional medicine, for the most part, takes a separative approach. It looks at and attempts to treat specific symptoms. I prefer the holistic approach. I view disease as the manifestation of blockages in the overall energy system in its most condensed form: the physical body.

Whatever diagnosis of disease you may have received, it really comes down to a lack of flow to the area concerned. If it's the pancreas, diabetes may result; if the heart, high blood pressure; if a pelvis out of alignment, Restless Leg Syndrome or fibroids. No matter what symptoms you are experiencing, getting to the root of the issue is the key and this is what Block Therapy does!

Body's infrastructure

Growing up, we were all told to sit up straight. We would listen in the moment, but before long, would fall back into our usual bad habits. What we didn't understand was how significant the practice of good posture is to lifelong health because it actually impacts our breath.

In Jordan B. Peterson's 12 Rules For Life, the very first rule is "STAND UP STRAIGHT WITH YOUR SHOULDERS BACK" – noteworthy in a book that offers a complete "Antidote to Chaos".

The body has certain foundations designed to support proper cellular alignment. As with everything in life, there is a right place — a home — for each and every cell . . . and there are trillions of cells. In a perfectly aligned body, every cell is comfortably at home. But through the constant force of gravity and unconscious habits, cells migrate away from home over time. No one has a perfectly aligned body. It requires effort.

As B.K.S. Iyengar says in his Light on the Yoga Sutras of Patanjali: "Perfection in an Asana is achieved when the effort to perform it becomes effortless and the infinite being within is reached."

What this means is that, once we establish the discipline necessary to support cellular alignment, it is easy to maintain. When the fascia system is properly fed and cleaned, the cells are energized and magnetically supported to remain upright and in their proper position. If we aren't conscious of our posture and breathing, we collapse into our internal space, pulling our cells away from their natural resting places. I call this cellular migration.

Imagine your child hanging on to your arm all day. After a while, you begin to feel the pulling and tension in your shoulder, and will adjust your stance to adapt to this external force. Imagine this as a constant. How would your body react and feel? How would you return to your pre-hanging state?

Now imagine a lifetime filled with such incidents, compounded by emotional and mental stress. Layer after layer, adhesions develop in your tissue to keep the cells where they are needed. By middle age (even younger for the generation that grew up with computers, tablets, and cell phones), chronic pain is the norm. This is the reality for most of us.

But there is an alternative.

As cells migrate, their relative alignment is constantly changing. The body is made to move - compress, extend, rotate. Just look at a yogi or a gymnast. You can see the body's amazing ability to contort and then go back to its original position. Problems arise when distorted postures are maintained for extended periods, creating compromised alignment.

The good news is that change can happen. Restoring space is the solution. This is what Block Therapy does and it starts with breathing.

At the center of the body, the diaphragm muscle is appropriately placed. It is central to our overall physical function. It is the ceiling to the abdominal organs and the floor to the heart and lungs. When it is working properly, it moves up and down like a pump. Essentially, it is the engine of life in the body. Understanding how to use this muscle is of paramount importance.

The majority of our oxygen receptors (called alveoli) lie at the base of the lungs. The lungs are cone shaped with the left containing two lobes, the right having three. Air enters through the nose or mouth, moves past the throat and into the main airway — the trachea. It then proceeds into two branches, the bronchi, one for each lung, from which smaller and smaller branches, called bronchioles, move out. These are the passageways to the alveoli, which absorb oxygen and release carbon dioxide and waste gases.

The bronchioles and alveoli look like an upside down oak tree in the lungs. Along with the greatest concentration of alveoli, there is also more blood at the base, because gravity pulls everything down. So this is where the real magic of breathing happens.

A complete inhalation pulls air to the base of the lungs for optimal absorption into the bloodstream, and a complete exhalation removes waste to keep the system clean. A study done in 2014 in Australia, proved that 84% of weight loss comes from proper exhalation. Imagine that.

What about the conventional weight loss rules? Don't they apply?

I can tell you that they didn't for me. I was starving myself, working out regularly, expending more calories than I was ingesting — but my body was only getting bigger and harder . . . not the goal. What I have come to learn through personal experience is that all those efforts come to nothing if you aren't using your diaphragm properly.

To get this mechanism working for you, you have to consciously exercise the muscle. Otherwise it becomes weak. The diaphragm is unique in that it is the only muscle that functions consciously or unconsciously. This means that if you aren't intentionally using it, it will still work. However, a weak diaphragm gives rise to a host of problems as it is the foundation of the ribcage. If not supported through proper posture and strengthened through conscious breathing, it succumbs to the weight of the ribcage. Compressed, it can only function partially, so the body begins to rely on its back-up breathing muscles (those of the upper chest).

If this becomes habit, those secondary muscles take control. They don't pull the air deeply enough into the lungs to reach the rich bed of alveoli, so absorption is limited. Similarly, they don't remove waste as effectively so cell toxicity increases.

Think of a balloon filled with air. It almost defies gravity. We have the ability to keep our cells in this magical state. But remember what happens to a balloon as the days pass. It starts to lose its buoyancy as it ages and becomes heavy and wrinkled. As the space inside the balloon diminishes, the container becomes denser until gravity claims it.

When you breathe *consciously* with the diaphragm, you feed the body up to six times the oxygen due to the greater amount of absorption. This keeps the cells in the body light, symmetrical, buoyant, and healthy; oxygen maintains the space within, ensuring that the channels for flow stay open. As long as every cell is receiving its required nutrients, it functions with ease. When you breathe unconsciously with the muscles of the upper chest, the cells lose that buoyancy. Like the aging balloon, they become deflated and heavy. The result is a collapsed body full of pain.

There are also emotional consequences. Try holding your breath for a minute. Feel the panic building inside your body. This is how your cells feel when you aren't feeding them properly. Anxiety is something all of us feel at one time or another, and for some it's a chronic condition. If you are a chronic chest breather, you are creating the ideal environment for it. In the body of a chronic chest breather, many cells have had their lines of communication closed by scar tissue and adhesions.

If only 20% of your cells are in direct communication with your brain, there is a lot of missing information. The transmission is full of static, the conversation garbled. Unable to confirm the messages, the brain must improvise, and relying on experience it resorts to memory.

If you pay attention to how your body reacts and responds to stimuli and events, you begin to see how this works. For me, revelation came through my Yoga teacher- training program.

Part of our training focused on self-observation - noticing how you respond to stimuli. As I progressed, my antennae were definitely tuning in on different levels and I was beginning to get control of my reactions. That brought with it a sense of calm as I learned to exhale the moment and emotion before choosing a response. Inevitably, my reactions became actions, which took away any lingering attachment to how I might make others feel.

Then I had a profound experience that awakened me to a deep-rooted anxiety.

I was walking in a mall and passed a man, who looked at me as he scowled (or so I thought). Immediately, my gut tightened. I lost my breath and I felt a flood of acid enter my belly. I took a moment to consider the situation and connected some dots.

The scowl reminded me of how my Dad would look at me when he was disappointed. As a child, like many of us, I longed for my Dad's approval. For the most part, I was the teacher's pet. I liked to perform to my best and to receive recognition when deserved; and I wanted it most from my Dad. Some of my worst childhood memories were of disappointing him. He had a look that let me know in no uncertain terms how he felt and that feeling of disconnection that came through a glance was accompanied by a shift in warmth. It had a deep impact.

Prior to glimpsing the passing stranger's expression, I had felt light and free; in an instant I was consumed by anxiety. And this wasn't even about me. Perhaps as I passed him he thought of something that made him unhappy and it was just a coincidence that our eyes locked in that moment. Or maybe he had an arthritic knee that gave him a jolt of pain as we made eye contact. The point is there are many possibilities . . . and who cares. I mean really, if a dude I don't know scowls at me for some reason, it really isn't my problem.

My ego was trapped in a moment and attached a story to the event, causing an internal change to my state of being. Most significantly, however, was the way my breath was tied directly to that anxious state. It only took a few focused exhalations to bring me back to the lightness of moments before, and with it came an overwhelming sense of gratitude for how I had learned to manage my anxiety.

That was the first time I realized that most of my issues are created in my own head from memories of the past. Each moment is unique in itself and how we choose to see it is something we can control. The more I awakened to the understanding of breathing life into your cells and listening to what they say, the more I removed myself from past memory. It was as though I was freeing myself from a prison of my own making.

Joe Dispenza, in <u>Evolve Your Brain</u>, describes this sensation perfectly in revealing questions: "[I]s it possible that the seemingly unconscious thoughts that run through our mind daily and repeatedly create a cascade of chemical reactions that produce not only *what* we feel but also *how* we feel? Can we accept that the long- term effects of our habitual thinking just might be the cause of how our body moves to a state of imbalance, or what we call disease? Is it likely, moment by moment, that we train our body to be unhealthy by our repeated thoughts and reactions?"

One of my clients, a 27-year-old male, suffered from acute anxiety disorder. Every uncertainty he encountered (and there were many) virtually paralyzed him with worry and doubt. He decided to start using the Block every day as a regular practice. After only a day he reported back to me excitedly that his entire attitude and outlook had changed. He was calmer and more relaxed. After that, though he would experience occasional relapses, just knowing the Block was there to help him would instantly restore his composure. Plainly, he had found a tool that enabled him to manage his disabling condition.

Life is what we make it. Living with anxiety, stress and depression is not fun. Of course life presents challenges to us all. It's not meant to be easy; we are here to learn and to grow. But no matter what your circumstances, opening your body to a fuller intake of oxygen will improve your outlook, your effectiveness, your very sense of who you are. It is a life-altering practice, and the equipment is "built in".

Concerns with infrastructure are also relevant to concerns with aging. When people talk about anti-aging, the face is usually the focal point of discussion. I love sharing the benefits of my work as it relates to keeping the face looking young because it's not about looking twenty when you are fifty; it's about keeping the cells positioned where they are supposed to be.

Real beauty is reflected in health. You can be superficially attractive, even striking, but beauty radiates from the eyes, the skin, the smile, and the heart. This is pretty hard to fake with makeup and surgeries. But let's get to the nitty-gritty of how Fluid Isometrics actually reverses time in your tissue.

I have mentioned before that every cell has its rightful place. As long as cells are in correct alignment, there is optimal space for blood and oxygen flow to reach them. Also, cells that are properly fed and clean actually glow because they aren't starving for nutrients and their light isn't blocked by toxins or built up residue. A person with healthy skin stands out in a crowd.

Aging ultimately is a product of gravity. We aren't aware that this force is constantly dragging our tissue down, so we don't try to counteract it. Yet there is an anti-aging mechanism built right into your body: the full conscious exhalation. It may sound far-fetched that proper breathing will make you look younger, but fully oxygenated cells look like a balloon full of air, as opposed to one only partially full sinking to the ground. Deflated cells are not uniform or balanced, so they look tired and heavy; this is what happens when they are starved of oxygen.

Conscious awareness of alignment is another anti-aging factor the majority of us fail to appreciate. Symmetry is fundamental to aesthetics; we see it recurring throughout nature. It embraces harmony, rhythm, and equilibrium. We are unconsciously drawn toward those things that appear symmetrical finding them naturally pleasing.

Most faces are asymmetrical because of our left/right side bias. The average person's head tilts either left or right, depending on which side is dominant. If you are always hanging your head to the left – a common posture for a right-handed person – then the fascia will be pulled down to the left affecting the alignment of your tissue.

Remember, the fascia is ingenious in its design and it is here to protect us. When there are forces acting on the cells, the fascia responds. If tissue starts to hang down because of poor foundation and breath, the fascia will hook onto the bone to keep those cells from falling further. These hooks are a double-edged sword: they defend us against immediate decline, but over time they block flow to other cells in the area. Cells deprived of blood and oxygen flow become heavy and dirty, adding more mass to the already sagging tissue. This becomes a vicious cycle.

Look at yourself in the mirror and note your head alignment. Which eye sits lower? Whichever one it is, notice how the jaw appears different on each side. The side that hangs lower will likely have excessive skin hanging as well. What about age spots? Any accumulation of color indicates an area of tissue where melanin has clumped together. Although sun damage is the known culprit for age spots, if the tissue had been fully spacious so the cells had optimal flow, melanin wouldn't have had the opportunity to settle and stick. Flow is the key, and with symmetry there is optimal flow.

Consider another example: the Charlie Brown Christmas tree. It was not the first choice because its branches weren't even and it looked kind of sad. If you see a butterfly with a broken wing, it doesn't stand out as a perfect specimen. The brain picks up on symmetry and notices when it isn't present. All the expensive creams in the world won't change what's going on under the surface, and, unfortunately, those surgeries that promise to make you look younger take your cells from one place of incorrect alignment and force them into another place where they don't belong.

Short term, this may appear to be an improvement; but long-term, the surgery will simply add more scar tissue, and we have already noted that scar tissue is really the source of pain, aging and disease.

Fascia decompression and Block Therapy are designed to release the hooks of fascia from the bone and inflate the cells with oxygen and keep them clean. Through foundation strengthening, the area of focus becomes balanced and symmetrical. This is a safe, natural and simple way to align your cells: feed them with the nutrients they need and support them in their alignment. When we do this for them, they do their job for us.

Focus on the heart muscle

Imagine a box packed full of tennis balls. Now imagine sitting on the box. What happens to the contents?

First of all, they shift from their positions as the container - the box - shifts in its alignment. The box may even break if the pressure exerted is great enough, and some of the balls may spill out, depending on how sturdy it is.

Structural heart disease refers to abnormalities of the heart's structure. And what is required for any structure to maintain its integrity? Space. The single most important thing your heart muscle needs is room to function.

The aorta is the main artery leaving the heart. It needs to be supported in proper alignment so the heart can send blood through it to feed all the cells in the body. The collapse of the rib cage into the core puts immense pressure on the heart and squeezes the aorta, forcing the heart muscle to work harder to get the job done.

The Block Therapy system is designed to promote heart health through, first, creating space in the tissue (in this case re-aligning the ribcage), and, second, strengthening the diaphragm muscle to both provide a continual massage to the heart through its pumping action, and support the heart with its strong and solid foundation. When the diaphragm is working efficiently, up to six times the oxygen is absorbed into the body, according to Stephen Cope in <u>Yoga and the Quest For the</u> <u>True Self.</u>

Once again, we must look at the foundation, the diaphragm, and the collapse of the rib cage, head, neck, and arms in an unconscious person, to see how alignment and proper breathing are crucial to heart health. Without awareness of these things, the collapse of the body over time will be the greatest contributor to structural heart disease, which traditional medical doctors frequently term as congestive heart failure (CHF), determined by when an image of the heart in an echocardiogram shows the muscle pumps a very small percentage rather than at or close to 100%.

Heart failure occurs when the heart is unable to pump sufficiently to maintain blood flow to meet the body's needs. Signs and symptoms of heart failure commonly include shortness of breath, excessive tiredness, and leg swelling. This is no surprise, being that the heart is designed to pump blood and oxygen to the cells.

Without this, the cells become starved and dirty.

Yet this is just a sped-up version of everybody's fate. This is what happens as we age, and what we ultimately die from if nothing else takes us beforehand. The heart simply doesn't have the strength to pump life to all cells indefinitely. At the end of life, the heart fails, and the body dies. This is a natural process, but it doesn't have to happen as early as the accepted norm.

If you believe what I say and can see a correlation between heart disease and unconscious posture and breathing, you should also see that you have far more control over what happens to you as you age than you think. Heart health requires the same understanding as cell health. Heart cells, like all other cells, need three things to thrive: space, breath, and proper temperature.

So, if you are facing or anticipating heart problems, consider using Block Therapy to address them. You may be able to slow down or even reverse the effects. It works if you do the work, and there is no other organ that needs your attention more than your heart.

Channel problems (vascular vulnerability)

Where regular uninterrupted flow is the basis of optimal health, in dealing with any compromises to flow, we must always look to the channels that convey it.

Two major problems with the body's channels are disease types named after their affected conduits: **Coronary Artery Disease** (involving the channels that take oxygen from the lungs to the body) and Coronary Vascular Disease (affecting the transport of waste gasses back to the lungs for exhalation). These conditions are caused by a hardening of the arteries (atherosclerosis), which happens when the arteries are narrowed or blocked, and weak or damaged veins (eg. varicose veins)

Diet and a sedentary lifestyle are usually blamed for this condition, which definitely makes sense; however, there is more to it than what you put in your mouth and whether or not you exercise in the traditional sense of the word.

Fats are really to blame here, based on the definition of what causes this disease. But let's look at fat and how it changes when heat is applied.

Butter at room temperature is a solid; heat it up and it quickly liquefies. If fat is creating plaque in the artery, taking away space for flow, it is because the fat is colder than the temperature required to melt it.

Back in the chapter on fascia and tissue temperature, we discussed how the cells should be at 98.6 degrees Fahrenheit for optimal health. Butter at this temperature would definitely be a liquid, but at room temperature, it's a solid. As an experiment, place your hands on your feet, or your outer thighs, or, for many of you, your abdomen, and notice the temperature. As I mentioned in my story, I used to come back from a five mile run dripping wet with sweat, yet my belly still felt cold. This was because there were so many blockages to flow.

Now place your hand on your left lower ribs. This is the area just below your heart and where the aorta is situated. Keeping the flow open here is of crucial importance for heart health. For this channel to be open and spacious, it must have no blockages, be properly heated to keep the fats that run through it liquid, and be structurally supported to keep the walls aligned and strong.

The challenge for many is that this is one of the first areas we collapse into our core. This is especially true of the right handed, who constitute the majority of the population.

So why does this affect your aorta?

Lift your right arm above your head and mimic throwing a ball. Go through the motion a few times. Notice what happens to the left lower ribs during the action. They compress repeatedly. For the right-handed person, the left lower rib cage is subject to this compressive action constantly.

It's simple mechanics. The rib cage is like an accordion that adjusts to provide range of motion and support.

Problems arise when the ribs are chronically compressed. If after each compressive action the body were reset to a neutral alignment, there wouldn't be an issue. But people simply aren't aware of this, and as a result an area of tissue becomes blocked due to repetitive negative postural actions, incorrect breathing, and a container that can't support optimal flow. It becomes cold, and the fats turn into a solid plaque.

This is why atherosclerosis occurs; but it can be undone by melting the adhesions, connecting to the diaphragmatic breath and understanding and practicing proper postural alignment.

Two other channel problems are aneurysm (when an artery bulges in a weak spot) and stroke (when it occurs in the brain). There are three types of stroke, but 87% of victims have what's called an ischemic stroke, which results from a lack of blood flow to the brain. The parts of the brain affected depends on what area is deprived of blood and oxygen. Once again, blockage is the culprit, so let's look at how keeping the fascia system aligned and healthy can prevent a stroke and even reverse some of the negative effects after one.

Noticeably prevalent in our society, especially with today's technology, is the forward tilted head. Correct alignment of head and shoulders would involve arms in line with shoulders, but this is rarely the case.

In the front of the neck are the carotid arteries. These are the main arteries that supply blood and oxygen to the head and brain. In order for optimal flow to occur, the channels need to be open. If there is plaque built up in the arteries, or compression on them, flow will be diminished.

Let's first look at how managing fascia health can prevent the build-up of plaque. We have discussed how plaque is made up of fats and cholesterol, and how certain temperatures are required for fats to be liquid. To have proper tissue temperature throughout the body requires that the diaphragm be working as it is the engine that keeps the cells heated. But the reality is that most people are breathing from the upper chest. This creates ideal conditions for a stroke.

First, when breathing doesn't arise from the diaphragm muscle, it becomes weak. The diaphragm is the foundation for the ribcage, its contents, and everything it supports: head, shoulders, arms . . . If this muscle declines, the ribcage collapses into the core of the body, pulling everything forward with it. Right behind the collarbones lie the carotid arteries. With forward head alignment, these arteries have a barricade putting immense pressure on the roadways, slowing the flow of blood and oxygen to the head.

What's more, the muscles of the upper chest end up doing the breathing, which isn't their job. They are designed to kick in when deeper breaths are required, but most people are chronically breathing with them. The result is that they become hard and dense from overuse, which puts even more pressure into this area, taking away even more space from the carotid arteries.

And on top of all this, the chest breather isn't capable of heating all parts of the body, as the diaphragm is the body's furnace. Breathing with the secondary muscles leaves the body cold, which creates an opportunity for fats to stick to the walls of the arteries, blocking blood and oxygen flow to the brain.

Attending to fascia health is a way to prevent, manage and potentially reverse some of the effects of a stroke. The body has tremendous powers of self-repair if the cells are given what they need. Our job is to open the channels for flow by melting any adhesions blocking the way, keeping the tissue heated through proper diaphragmatic breathing, and strengthening the foundations to support cell alignment.

I have been working with a gentleman who had a stroke eight years prior to our meeting. He was paralyzed on his right side; his right arm and leg had no feeling or movement. He was able to walk with a cane/walker, but was supporting his entire weight on his left side, pulling his right side through momentum as he propelled himself forward. He also was unable to talk. His cognitive function was still high, but his vocabulary was limited to five words.

Before his stroke, he had been a drummer. I can only imagine the frustration one feels in a body that doesn't respond to one's wishes. To have been a musician, an artist, an athlete, living for one's passion and have had that taken away . . . To exist in one's body, unable to move at will, or say what one wants to say . . .

I had been working with the man for seven months, only seeing him on average twice a month. What was amazing was that he was so willing to do whatever he could to assist the process. I was doing Fluid Isometrics on him, and he was managing to use the block at home, in between treatments, to the best of his ability. Because he couldn't mobilize one side of his body, even positioning the block was often challenging.

The most obvious area of concern for him when I started was his leg. Walking had caused a great deal of pain in the joints of his right leg because he would use that leg as a splint to stay mobile, which was adding up to increasing soreness in the foot and knee. There was also so much compression and twisting in the leg that the foot itself had virtually no blood flow. It was hard and cold with no signs of life, a contracted mess.

When I first met him, I knew there was a lot of work to do, but he had the will and we had the time. In the beginning, progress was slow. We were starting with a body that had seized into a state of injury eight years old; it was frozen in that contracture and alignment, and it would take some time to get it heated enough to make significant changes.

We proceeded, and as the months passed, I noticed with excitement the signs of gradual regeneration. His right foot started to come to life: blood vessels appeared, where before, the flesh had looked like a blue, frozen mass; the tissue got warmer and softer: and the foot was planting on the ground with better connection. But it was the work in the core and rib cage that brought about the most substantial developments. And one momentous day, I realized we had hit a new level.

I hadn't seen him for three weeks. The previous treatment I had felt was a game changer. We had spent our time in the pelvis, core and ribcage, and brought what I felt was a new sense of openness and balance to his body. When I entered his room at this next appointment, he received me with excitement and an eagerness to explore.

At first, I didn't know what he was telling me, given his five-word vocabulary. Seeing that I wasn't grasping his point, he walked over and grabbed his iPad. In it he had homework to help him with his language and writing skills. He showed me that his scores were improving, and he was getting better at his cognitive challenges.

Thrilled to see this, I was chomping at the bit to dive back into our work. Once he was set, his exuberance even greater than usual, he said a new word.
I couldn't believe my ears. I asked him if this was a new thing he could do since our last treatment. He nodded yes, which inspired me further to get right to work and continue to open his body. What unfolded toward the end of that treatment shocked and awed me . . . and I'm not easily shocked and awed.

His right arm was typically incredibly bound and frozen. Anatomical position, the natural resting alignment of the perfect body, would have the palms facing forward when standing. If you look at anyone walking around, the palms are facing back as an indication of how far we are from correct alignment.

His right arm was so frozen in internal rotation that when he was lying on his back, the arm wouldn't stay where you positioned it. Rather, it would spring back to the "stroke" alignment and if I tried to force it, there would be obvious pain. When we met for that day's treatment, he had also shared that he felt pain in his right bicep.

When blood and oxygen flow infiltrate tissue previously blocked, generally the first thing a person experiences is pain as the nerve fibers are waking up. This "new" awareness I compare to opening your eyes in the morning and having the stinging sensation of light entering your vision before you are ready for that influx. It can feel painful until you adapt.

Throughout the treatment, I was working deep in his belly to address the psoas muscle and bring more balance and awareness in the gut. I also spent time on his ribcage and throat as well as working in the right arm to open the channels for even greater flow. At one point, focused on his right elbow, I felt a shifting of the joint, immediately sensing more life in his hand.

Approaching the end of the session, I felt there had been a significant adjustment, and I simply wanted to connect to his right palm and fingers. Placing the back of his hand in my left hand, and taking my right hand to his palm, I started to apply pressure with the patterned technique to open the channels. Remember, he had been a drummer. This is where it gets interesting.

So imagine: he is lying flat and I am sitting on his right side. I have his right hand cupped in my hands. His body is sweating from the work, an indicator of positive change. All at once, he starts lifting his right leg up toward the ceiling and bringing it back down, in a continual repetitive cycle, with his left hand and arm moving in rhythm, as though he were drumming.

Startled at first by the aggressiveness of the movements, I asked him if he was doing this on purpose. He said no, and kept looking at me in awe and saying, "Wow!!!!!" I soon realized that he was connected to a time when he had been performing. He even added in the beat and rhythm with his voice. This went on for about five minutes and the delight for me was in seeing his core engaging in a symmetrical manner as his body responded to this primal urge inside of him.

We finished the session and I had him sit upright. In that instant our incredible breakthrough was affirmed. Until then, his right side had been a burden to his movements, evident in the awkward way he carried himself. Now all that had changed. Sitting up, he moved with greater ease than before. The frozen tissue had awakened; in fact, it radiated strength and power.

Body Electronics

Another significant form of disease involves the channels that transmit nervous impulses. These may be compared to the wiring in an electrical system.

With arrhythmia, the electrical impulses to the heart are interrupted. There are many factors that can cause heart rhythm disorders - stress being one of them. But let's look at how incorrect posture and unconscious breathing also play a role.

The diaphragm muscle is the floor to the heart muscle. Like with any foundation, if it is weak, it can't support what rests on top of it. When you aren't a conscious breather, this foundation becomes weak, full of scar tissue, and unable to generate the internal heat required for electrical impulses to flow.

On top of this, if proper alignment of the ribcage, head, neck, and arms isn't considered and practiced, the weight of these structures pushes down on the heart, adding extra pressure to it. This affects the flow of everything to the heart - including electrical impulses.

Early in my career, before I even understood this, I was treating a woman with a frozen shoulder. As the ribcage is the foundation for the shoulder joint, this area became the focus of her treatment. I worked on her every week for six weeks. On the day of her last treatment, she shared that not only was her shoulder pain gone and range of motion restored, but that her arrhythmia (a problem she had not even mentioned), had gone away. I suddenly realized in one of those flashes of intuition that the pressure on her ribcage that we had removed had been the cause of the other condition.

In addition to irregular heartbeats that are linked to stress and electric impulse irregularities, another neuro-impulse disease is Alzheimer's. It happens when plaques containing beta amyloid (sticky proteins that accumulate outside nerve cells) form in the brain, causing inflammation that damages neurons. This blocks neural transmissions and affects cognitive function. But just as with plaques in the aorta or carotid arteries, preventing the buildup would also prevent the symptoms.

We have yet to discover a cure for Alzheimer's, but keeping the fascia system healthy is an effective deterrent.

Years ago I had the opportunity to work with a gentleman suffering from severe Alzheimer's. When I first met him, what was strikingly obvious was his distorted head and neck alignment. His resting head posture had him staring at the floor. When I spoke to his wife about this, she mentioned that every day he would fall asleep in a chair, head hanging forward. I saw this as a major culprit in the onset of his condition. Unfortunately, by the time I began his treatments, he was limited in his capacity and no change to this daily posture was introduced. That's the thing about the fascia — you need to be an active participant in your own healing to get results.

The body is ingenious in its design. As I have said before, I see inflammation as a priceless healing agent for cell repair. But, if we don't assist it, it accumulates, adding pressure to the afflicted area, becoming stagnant and acidic, a breeding ground for disease.

The body sends increased blood flow to where the cells need attention. Whether the area is stressed from injury, or blocked due to compression, the body knows how to deal with the damage: through inflammation. What we need to do is to support this healing process by giving the area more energy. Most often, with inflammation comes pain. With pain comes fear, and this affects how we breathe; in fact, it causes us to reactively hold the breath, which is the opposite of what needs to be done. Getting the diaphragmatic breath working strongly on our behalf as well as applying practices that improve flow and support cell alignment, is how we can help inflammation do its job to rebuild and heal.

It all comes back to the basics of keeping your fascia system healthy. Of course, prevention is the best approach, but even if right action is taken after disease arises, as long as a person can connect to conscious breath, healing can occur.

Hormone fluctuations

Here again I have a problem with the conventional approach, which treats an impaired function by artificially adding in a missing ingredient. My treatment is to stimulate the affected organs to get them working properly and producing what is needed.

The most frequently diagnosed and considered hormonal issue that stretches across genders is diabetes, both insulin-dependent and non-insulin dependent types. Diabetes is on the rise, and the number of people affected globally is staggering. Some of the conditions this disease can lead to are blindness, kidney failure, heart attack, stroke, and limb amputation. Needless to say, getting a hold on the situation in advance is far better than dealing with a condition after it arises.

There are two types of diabetes, the most common being Type 2 (when the body doesn't effectively use insulin to control blood sugar). Poor diet and sedentary lifestyle are major culprits, and child obesity is making this issue increasingly common in the young.

On that note, it was already stated that 84% of weight loss occurs through proper exhalation, as we saw in the Medical News Study done in Australia in 2014. This alone tells us that if the increase in diabetes is related to weight gain and obesity, then proper diaphragmatic breathing would be a major asset in the prevention of the disease.

The pancreas (the organ which secretes insulin) is situated in the center of the body, right below the diaphragm muscle. This is another reason why learning to breathe from the diaphragm would be beneficial - it would help to keep this organ healthy. Using this muscle regularly would give the pancreas a continual massage, maintaining sufficient blood and oxygen flow to keep it fed and clean. As long as cells are fed and clean, they are doing their job; in this case, secreting insulin to control blood sugar.

Finally, keeping the foundation strong with correct posture to prevent the collapse of the ribcage and everything else above, would take tremendous pressure off the organ, giving it the room it needs to function.

I have been working with a 62-year-old diabetic male who, when diagnosed, absolutely rejected insulin treatment. Instead, he chose to try my approach, combined with appropriate diet change. Within a short period of time, he had lost weight and was showing a remarkable drop in his blood sugar levels. His condition continues to improve.

Another example of hormonal-related injury that isn't as well understood by traditional medicine experts is fibromyalgia, which is commonly triggered by traumatic events or injury, and is often seen in adults who had a challenging and abusive childhood.

Symptoms may include widespread musculoskeletal pain, mood issues, and problems with memory, sleep, and fatigue.

This comes as no surprise given what we have seen earlier. Pain, fear, and stress cause us to reactively hold the breath. If these conditions persist for prolonged periods, or if a trauma or accident occurs that puts the body into a freeze response, the cells become starved for oxygen, and the lack of flow in the tissue results in toxicity.

When oxygen isn't reaching the cells, pain and fatigue set in, as the body is working but not getting the food it needs to sustain it. The brain even requires oxygen to fall into deep sleep, required for rejuvenation and healing. If the body is depleted, it's tired, it hurts, and you certainly won't be in a good mood.

I have worked with many who suffer from fibromyalgia and those who put the time in get the benefits. Strengthening the diaphragmatic breath and opening the flow to the cells not only releases toxins accumulated, but also awakens the stagnant inflammation to its healing potential. Repair occurs and the body reaps the benefits of renewal. This in turn improves the individual's overall outlook and mood, as pain and fatigue diminish.

Some people question whether fibromyalgia is real. I personally don't view the body as having disease, but rather barricades to blood and oxygen flow. Whatever cells are starved will scream with pain; it's simply the language they use to let us know they need attention. If that pain is widespread, it means there are many cells throughout the body that are blocked from life. Melting through adhesions in fascia and strengthening diaphragmatic breathing is a solution to the misery/mystery of fibromyalgia.

RETURNING TO THE BEGINNING

Fascia and Pregnancy

I don't have kids, so I don't pretend to know what it's like to be pregnant. However, what I do know is that space is required for health. When you are nurturing life in your belly, having the room to expand as the fetus grows is essential to a healthy birth.

So what does this mean? Returning to Stephen King's IT: the teenagers in the first version were each physically unique, but uniformly their cores had space. Like me, they didn't grow up in front of computers and while their bodies were not perfect by any means, they were open and spacious. Compare that to today's youth, habituated to computers and cell phones . . . their bodies are markedly different.

Try this. Sit in a chair, feet flat on the floor, knees bent 90 degrees, and lean back. Put your hands on your belly and notice that between the ribcage and the pelvis, there is space. Now lose the conscious connection and slump as most people do when sitting. Notice how much closer the ribcage is to the pelvis. This slumped posture starts much younger today. For girls, its consequence is less space in the belly to grow new life.

If you grew up before technology took its toll, you have the advantage of being able to assume upright posture at will. You can't maintain it indefinitely as the fascia will eventually pull you back down, but you can manage it for a good period of time.

Not so the current generation. They didn't start with space they then lost slowly over the years; they settled into a slumped posture early in life, blocking their natural diaphragmatic breath, causing collapse and adhesions. By the time they are ready to create life, their bellies are so compressed and gummed up that their capacity to expand as the fetus grows is impaired.

Adhesions in the core aren't linear. One side of the belly will always be more compressed than the other because we are dominant on one side, which creates natural asymmetry. This alone can evoke the potential for scoliosis in a child as limited tissue expansion can alter symmetrical growth. Any adhesions in the area will restrict natural expansion and impede the growing fetus.

Also, a developing baby adopts the breathing pattern of the mother. Young women are now more out of touch with their diaphragm than ever. This is a problem. I have worked with many babies who aren't breathing diaphragmatically (I will dive deeper into this shortly).

We of the older generations at least started out breathing with the belly; then, over the years through pain, fear and stress, we began reactively holding the breath, changing where it came from to the muscles of the upper chest.

I know this sounds scary, and for those who don't find a solution, there will be multiple challenges. However, if you are reading this, you have been drawn to a solution that is simple and highly effective - and anyone can change an existing situation at any time.

I repeat: you can improve your fascia health, at any age, no matter what your condition. As long as you have conscious awareness of your body and breath, applying the Block Therapy process will bring about positive change.

So back to the mother of today: unless you are having babies later in your years, you are coming from a place of decreased space in your belly. If you have the goal of getting pregnant, creating space now would be the best way to prepare your body to grow a healthy baby.

Also, if you have already had a child, the Block Therapy process will help to heal your belly from the trials of pregnancy. Remember what we said about stretch marks in relation to bodybuilding. The same stresses apply to the abdomen during pregnancy, creating in that area the same sort of scar tissue.

On another note, many couples are having trouble conceiving. The compressed pelvis and abdomen have tons of adhesions and scar tissue. For women, this can manifest as an inability to release an egg for fertilization during ovulation. For men, the symptoms may be depressed sperm motility, or even erectile dysfunction, which is becoming more prevalent at an earlier age.

Either way, the parents-to-be are working with reproductive equipment that has been compromised by the posture of technology. This is hampering a couple's ability to create a child in the first place and challenging the health of the child once born.

Dealing with the matter properly right from the start is the best way to ensure a healthy pregnancy, delivery, and future life for everyone involved.

Fascia and Babies

For those of you who have brought life into the world, you now have a little one who will rely on you for everything for a while. This is a special time for you, and there are simple things you can do to ensure that your baby has a body that functions well. This also helps you, because a healthy baby sleeps well.

Today, many babies are born with incorrect breath. Their little bodies that require oxygen as the main nutrient to grow and thrive are markedly depleted, causing major issues right from day one, but consciously aware parents can help their babies develop breathing correctly from day one.

Good breathing is essential to sound growth and development. Because most of you having babies at this time grew up physically distorted by technology, your child will be handicapped when it comes to full and complete diaphragmatic breath. This shouldn't be taken lightly, as all development from this point forward is dependent on the amount of oxygen each cell receives.

The good news is that because babies are light and adaptable, they can be carried around easily. Even better is the fact that the body wants to function as it designed. This means that if we give a body what it needs to do its job, it easily integrates the work and creates positive habits to sustain its requirements. And with babies, their bodies naturally respond to any stimuli that will take them back to their roots.

The simple act of applying consistent, controlled, and balanced pressure into the rib cage will give the child the opportunity to reconnect with its diaphragmatic breath.

No one realizes the significance of this. It means better sleep, digestion, and processing of all baby's bodily functions . . . which in turn means better sleep for you!

Years ago, I started working with a one-year-old girl. They believed she might have had a stroke in the womb. When I first met her, she wasn't able to move at all on her own. She had never crawled or even rolled over from her back. My immediate suspicion on being told of her condition had been that she didn't have any connection to her diaphragm.

It was so interesting because I could feel the lack of blood and oxygen flow in her tissue. Her legs felt spongy and dry, almost brittle. Also, from her working her muscles in the upper chest to breathe, her neck protruded forward and her eyes looked as though they were bugging out (this last due to the immense internal pressure inside her little body).

I worked with her for about a year and we made exciting gains. My focus was on getting her diaphragm to function so she could start to oxygenate her cells. In time, her body began to respond. Her appearance changed and her eyes grew smaller. Her head began to migrate back to a more aligned position. As her diaphragm took over from her upper chest, a more relaxed flow was emerging.

It was also obvious from the texture of her legs that life was awakening in her cells and during our time together, she began to walk. A couple of years ago, her mom sent a picture of her, saying she was an active, happy little girl. There has been some learning impairment, but from the perspective of her initial state, the difference the work made to her body and resultant quality of life was like night and day.

As I have said, the technique is simple. The parents must learn how to activate the proper breath as the magic lies in the daily work. It requires little time, and virtually no skill; just knowing how to apply pressure to heat up the ribcage and release the diaphragm muscle. The body wants to function as it is designed, but if it is frozen, it can't. As in starting the car on a cold day, sometimes you have to jump start the engine, then let it run awhile before you drive. A muscle in deep freeze is no different, and for a baby breathing with the muscles of the upper chest that is exactly the state of the diaphragm.

Fascia and Toddlers

Some parents may be reading this when their children are two to five years old - not babies anymore, but not in a position to do Block Therapy themselves (there is a Block for Kids Program that I recommend you begin at about age six). For this younger age bracket, we offer a series that teaches parents how to align and open the ribcage for the child.

We must keep pace with a changing world. Parents who have grown up with technology are having kids with unprecedented physical challenges. If we can recognize this, we can take action to ensure them a healthy future. Otherwise, they will be older in their bodies than their parents — not a pleasant thought.

I have been encountering a growing number of toddlers with issues reflective of a misaligned rib cage – specifically, problems with their hands, like cysts and trigger finger. I never used to see this in patients at such a young age.

The diaphragm is the foundation of the ribcage and when functioning properly, it moves up and down in the core. This creates a strong platform for the shoulder joints, head, and neck; when the breath is strong, the foundation is balanced and reasonably symmetrical. Time after time, meeting these kids, I can see immediately that their rib cages are not aligned. As with an accordion, when one side compresses, the other balloons. If this is the actual alignment of the child's rib cage, the foundation for the shoulder blades will be off, causing each arm to track differently.

When the shoulder blades can't properly track, it affects the alignment all the way down the chain to the fingertips. It's one thing if this happens once we have fully grown; it's another if your baby or toddler is that far out of alignment to start. Growing up misaligned makes for a far more challenging life path.

As with babies, it's all about melting through the adhesions in the ribcage. The body wants to breathe from the right place. No skill is required to initiate this process; just a knowledge of how to position the ribcage and how long to maintain pressure to get the desired heating effect. This, in turn, changes the way the shoulders, arms and hands move and function as well as improving blood and oxygen flow to the head, neck, brain, and everything else in that region.

Five minutes per day is all it takes to change your child's life. This sounds dramatic, and it is. We don't see changes happening if they are constant and gradual. If you lost twenty pounds over the course of a year, you likely wouldn't see it until someone else mentioned it. Because you see your kids every day, you don't notice how different they look compared to kids when you were a child.

But there is a blessing in disguise here because the earlier a person embraces the conscious diaphragmatic breath, the better life will be. Helping your child make this a habit is a gift whose value is beyond measure.

OUR FURRY FRIENDS

J ust as fascia connects all the cells in the human body, so it does in all other animals.

I had my first experience working on a dog many years back, and it was incredible. She was an older lap dog; you could tell from the way she walked and moved that she had lost the vigor of youth.

I had her resting on my lap, her body cradled in my hands with my palms applying balanced pressure to her body. She seemed to love this pressure, as she allowed me to hold her without squirming.

As with a human body, I picked up her flow and slowly started to move my hands in her fascia. I wasn't rubbing the surface; but moving between the layers of fascia as her body accepted my pressure. To an observer, it would have looked like a dance: I was rocking slowly in my seat, left to right, as I rhythmically followed her flow, and she surrendered in the most beautiful way.

It was fun to see the expression of her owner (also a patient of mine). She was looking at me in awe, surprised that her little love would permit this manipulation. We worked together this way for about twenty minutes until she was let down onto the ground.

She immediately started running around with astonishing energy. Her owner said to me, "She hasn't moved like that in years." It was like she was a playful puppy again. That was when I first realized that fascia is fascia and the body intuitively knows what it needs.

Since then I haven't spent a lot of time with pets, as I have made work with people my priority, but this past summer I had the opportunity to work with a beautiful gentle giant.

My friend, Heather, who also works with me, has a beautiful backyard with a pool, so we decided that on Fridays during the summer, whenever possible, we would hang out together, enjoying the beautiful weather. She has a huge dog named Marley – a cross between a shepherd and a Great Dane.

Shepherds often have issues with their hips, and Marley, at nine years old, was no exception – she was limping by the time I started working with her. Her left hip was the problem. Watching her walk from behind, I could see the joint collapsing into her body, causing the limp.

I mentioned that we could do Fluid Isometrics on Marley, and that I believed we could get her to stop limping. I worked on her three times; then Heather took over, working on her daily.

Seeing this beautiful animal surrender to the work was exhilarating. The first treatment lasted about fifteen minutes; during that time, I worked with her on her side, her affected hip facing up. With the exception of a few friendly nips to let me know I was getting too close to her edge of discomfort, she lay there and allowed me to go quite deep.

I knew when she had had enough when her 120-pound frame stood up and walked away; but she was already moving with more freedom. A bit later, I spent some time working on her standing, getting my hands deep into the joint. She really enjoyed this, until she had reached her limit, but again she walked off with a better stride.

She even bounded down the stairs, shocking Heather, as before she would have done this more cautiously.

The next week we continued.

Heather's house is on a cul-de-sac, and when I pulled up in the driveway, Marley ran to the fence and gave me some of her "hello" barks. When I got to the backyard and met Heather, she said, "Wow, Marley gave you a love bark". As if I would know the difference, but her Mama did, and Marley obviously was excited to see me so she could have some more work done.

That day we only spent about twenty minutes, and I focused more on her back and hip to address the cause and pain sites, as in a human body. My reference to energy moving in waves and spirals are important, as this is the basis of the technique - moving in the same direction as the energy. What was noteworthy here was that you could see the energy spiral patterns (energy cysts) in her fur. The texture of the fur and her beautiful coloring made it easy to discern where time and attention were needed. Again, after the work, she moved with greater ease and confidence, bounding down the stairs, and playing more like a puppy according to Heather.

The third and last time I worked on her was unforgettable. Remember, this beautiful beast weighs 120 pounds. It's not like I could get her to do something she didn't want to do. When she lay down, it was on her bad hip, her left side, so I had to approach her from a different angle. I put my hand on the inside of her left hip and applied pressure straight down, which was really helpful, as it allowed me to move her hip toward the outside of her body (remember, it was collapsing into her body). As soon as I did this, she threw back her head, let out a big moan, and smiled. In that moment I fell in love with her. She let me continue with my work and didn't mind at all, until she had had enough and got up. We played with her, and again Heather remarked on how different she was in her energy and mobility.

The rest of the summer was busy, and I didn't have time to go there, so Heather took over and started working on her regularly. When we spoke about Marley in the fall, she shared how Marley was a completely new dog. She was happier. Only a year prior, she had been depressed due to the death of her sister. Now she had come out of her shell and demonstrated a sense of joyous freedom in her body. It was heartwarming to hear that this beautiful creature had become a loveable pup again.

At this stage in my career I find it necessary to focus on treating people. In the future, however, I intend to pursue this rich and rewarding application of Fluid Isometrics more fully.

Human or animal, we are all made up of fascia. Connect to the wisdom of this system and you have what you need to unzip the seams of time; to open the body to renewed life.

WHERE WE GO FROM HERE

Whatever your spiritual orientation - God, your higher self, the divine, your angels, the universe - your soul speaks through space. When you are compressed and stuck, your heart is trapped in a pattern that challenges flow. When you allow free and open flow, you connect to your wisdom and speak with truth. Perfection is never the goal; authenticity in the moment always is.

Being true to your misgivings, imperfections, and failures as well as your talents, passions, and beliefs will help you navigate the tides and surf the waves. Being in the flow of your existence is the most fulfilling way to live. It may be different from what you imagined, but your heart will know; your cells and fascia will support you on your journey. Getting you to the wisdom of your cells is the essence of Fluid Isometrics and Block Therapy. It is the bridge between your consciousness and your physical being.

We have an entire universe to discover; yet we have only scratched the surface of what is possible in this life. Everyday science is uncovering deeper layers of understanding of how the mind and body work, how we can manifest the reality we desire. It was only about a decade ago that science believed the brain was not regenerative. If you had a stroke, what was left was the best bet. If you killed brain cells from partying too much, they were lost forever. Today, we know this is not the case. I have seen first hand many times that our potential for healing is virtually limitless.

Let's shift our perspective and think of the body this way: the cells exist to support the fascia. This is how I see it, not the other way around. It is the fascia system that is the conscious container of the soul and the role of the cells is to provide what the fascia needs. We have given so much time and attention to understanding the cells' needs that we have missed what most requires our attention.

In his book <u>Successful Aging</u>, Daniel Levitin comments that the prefrontal cortex is susceptible to age-related decreases in blood flow, changes in the structure of cells, reduction of volume (shrinkage). A biological explanation is there is no evolutionary pressure for the prefrontal cortex to stay sharp in old age, just as there is no evolutionary pressure for anything to stay sharp in old age. And so processing speed, led by prefrontal cortex decline, slows down."

I have a different view.

The prefrontal cortex is the area of the brain located just behind the forehead. This brain region has been implicated in planning complex cognitive behavior, personality expression, decision-making, and moderating social behavior. The "shrinkage" that Daniel mentions in his book comes from compression as a result of the body tipping forward, which happens with normal aging. However, we have the ability to change the unconscious migration of the body toward the earth, to utilize the full diaphragmatic breath, and then strengthen proper foundations, to counter this unconscious habit.

In <u>Evolve Your Brain</u>, Joe Dispenza mentions, "The frontal lobe, when fully activated, gives us the capability to be much more in control of who we want to become than we probably realize. To break free from our emotional addictions, we must put the king back in the throne."

Once again, I see that in order to "put the king back in the throne", we must give the brain the space it needs to receive blood and oxygen. It all comes back to the same point: look after your fascia and you will thrive.

We have been too entangled in looking outside ourselves for answers. The answers are inside of us. The key is to learn the language of your cells because they are here to support the fascia. When you spend time lying on the Block, connecting to your sensations and breathing space into your compression, you are in direct communication with your higher self. This work is all about creating space. In doing so, you wring out the countless layers of environment that you have absorbed in your lifetime. Your fascia has stored it all and that is what causes you to age.

By meeting those environments with the Block Buddy, you open a door into yourself, let out what has been locked away, and exhale it. It isn't scary, it's liberating. Freeing yourself from the past is the only way to be present and allow the future to unfold in a peaceful and loving way. Just think of a world where everyone is at peace within. Impossible?

I don't think so. I see that we are moving into a new time. Because things are so fast paced, people are getting older at a younger age. But information is also spreading more quickly to those who search. As

Block Therapy achieves wider recognition, those who practice it will create an evolved state of fascia - one that will empower the body to thrive, rather than merely survive.

This will change the way people feel inside, and in turn the way they view the world. That's all it takes: more people making better choices. That will add up, elevating the world frequency, until love and compassion rule all decisions . . . someday.

This is my dream.

Breathe & Believe

ACKNOWLEDGMENTS

This book is the product of decades of struggle, service, and solidarity. I owe a debt of gratitude to everyone who has helped me on my journey.

To my many clients over the years who have come to me with their challenges and allowed me to work with them, my undying thanks. You gave me the opportunity to explore and develop my initial intuitions through invaluable practice.

I could not have achieved my dream of sharing this understanding with the world without my community and my team. Fluid Isometrics and Block Therapy are a work in progress, continually enhanced by the contributions of everyone involved. Thank you all.

Even the most prolific organization could not hope to survive in today's global market without solid backing, business experience, and legal knowledge. Thank you, Barry Shenkarow and Tim Dewart; your faith, guidance and support have been the life breath of our enterprise.

Writing a book is a vast endeavor in itself. Trish Field gave me the courage to proceed when I was still struggling to find my voice, generously bestowing her insight and experience. Michelle Vandepas of Gracepoint Publishing opened her doors and provided a home for this project. Heather Hillard brought the manuscript together in masterful form. As always, Reid Edwards, my first draft editor, gave me the freedom to let my thoughts flow onto paper, assured that they would emerge from the funnel of his grammatical discipline true to their essence. Finally, Dr. John Daugherty, with his consummate foreword, has given me validation that I have long been seeking. Thank you all from the bottom of my heart.

RESOURCES AND FURTHER INFORMATION

Cope, Stephen, *Yoga and the Quest for the True Self.* New York: Penguin Random House, 2000.

Dispenza, Joe, *Evolve Your Brain: The Science of Changing Your Mind.* Deerfield Beach, Florida: Health Communications Inc., 2007.

Iyengar, B.K.S., *Light on the Yoga Sutras of Patanjali.* Hammersmith: Thorsons, 2002. Levitin, Daniel, *Successful Aging.* Toronto: Penguin Random House Canada, 2020.

McIntosh, James, "Majority of Weight Loss Occurs 'Via Breathing'." *Medical News Today:* 2014: https://www.medicalnewstoday.com/articles/287046

Peterson, Jordan, B. *12 Rules for Life: An Antidote to Chaos.* Toronto: Random House Canada, 2018.

Tolle, Eckhart, *The Power of Now: A Guide to Spiritual Enlightenment.* Vancouver: Namaste Publishing, 2001.

To see Christopher's journey and transformation around scoliosis treatment — https://www.youtube.com/watch?v=FiaEfEjcRDo&t=126s

Listen to Edna's story on her own healing as well as leading others to healing with sharing the work in her native language — Discussions with the Fascia Masters: https://www.youtube.com/watch?v=Bc4jx-Pw7MX4&t=2772s

See how a Jones' Fracture treatment can work through Joe's progress — https://www.youtube.com/watch?v=ZEFK0RdugUM&t=4s

Watch how bone fractures can be healed through the professional sports injury interaction — https://www.youtube.com/watch?v=QeRmbrc5FXk

ABOUT THE AUTHOR

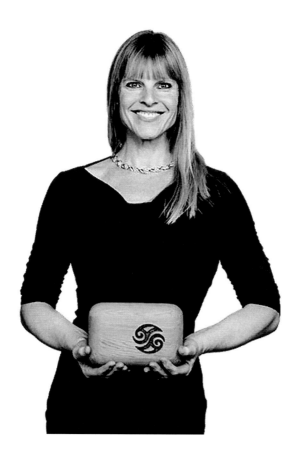

Deanna Hansen is a certified Athletic Therapist and the founder of Fluid Isometrics and Block Therapy, both techniques targeting the fascia system. She has been developing these principles for twenty years.

Her personal journey began around the age of thirty, with her body being decades older from years of abuse when younger. She suffered from addiction, anxiety, and depression; 50 pounds overweight, compacted, and twisted she awoke to a realization that she had to make a change during an anxiety attack.

Countering some unseen force within, Hansen was able to reach within her gut and let out a gasp of pent-up emotion, thus beginning a discipline that immediately changed her whole being. Not only was her physical self getting younger when she started applying techniques to the fascia, but her outlook on everything shifted.

Her methods help transform people on all levels and she is excited for you to embrace the breath within yourself.

Find out more about Block Therapy by visiting Deanna on the web at https://blocktherapy.com/.

QUANTUM LIVING

PRESS

Read other great books about health and healing by visiting www. gracepointpublishing.com.

Made in United States
North Haven, CT
21 June 2022

20435416R00074